COLOR ATLAS OF
CUTANEOUS EXCISIONS AND REPAIRS

This full-color atlas presents an in-depth pictorial display of cutaneous surgery designed for all those interested in improving their surgical skills, from students and residents to experienced surgeons across a wide range of medical specialties. It provides step-by-step instructions through a series of more than 400 detailed color photographs, including supplementary illustrations demonstrating appropriate techniques.

The excisions and resulting defects featured within, although primarily centered around the head and neck, cover a variety of locations. The repairs vary in type and size in order to provide multiple options in reconstruction. The chapters are separated into anatomic regions such as the eyelid, the ear, and the scalp, allowing the reader easy access to specific anatomic defects.

This atlas is the culmination of the years of experience gained by the authors in the surgical management of skin cancers.

COLOR ATLAS OF CUTANEOUS EXCISIONS AND REPAIRS

Ken K. Lee, MD

Director of Dermatologic Surgery
Associate Professor of Dermatology, Surgery, Otolaryngology/Head & Neck Surgery
Oregon Health & Science University
Portland, Oregon

Neil A. Swanson, MD

Professor and Chair, Department of Dermatology
Professor of Surgery, Otolaryngology/Head & Neck Surgery
Oregon Health & Science University
Portland, Oregon

Han N. Lee, MD

Director of Dermatologic Surgery, Assistant Professor of Dermatology
University of Southern California
Los Angeles, California

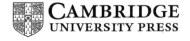
CAMBRIDGE
UNIVERSITY PRESS

CAMBRIDGE UNIVERSITY PRESS
Cambridge, New York, Melbourne, Madrid, Cape Town, Singapore, São Paulo, Delhi

Cambridge University Press
32 Avenue of the Americas, New York, NY 10013-2473, USA

www.cambridge.org
Information on this title: www.cambridge.org/9780521860246

First published 2008

Printed in India by Replika

A catalog record for this publication is available from the British Library.

Library of Congress Cataloging in Publication Data

Lee, Ken K., 1964–
Color atlas of cutaneous excisions and repairs / Ken K. Lee, Neil A. Swanson, Han N. Lee.
p. ; cm.
Includes bibliographical references and index.
ISBN 978–0–521–86024–6 (hardback)
1. Skin–Surgery–Atlases. I. Swanson, Neil A. (Neil Axel), 1949– II. Lee, Han N., 1970– III. Title.
[DNLM: 1. Reconstructive Surgical Procedures–methods–Atlases.   2. Skin–surgery–Atlases.   3. Skin
Transplantation–methods–Atlases. WR 17
L478c 2007]
RD520.L427 2007
617.4'77–dc22   2007022788

ISBN 978-0-521-86024-6 hardback

To our patients

Contents

Preface

This atlas presents an in-depth pictorial display of cutaneous surgery designed for all those interested in improving their surgical skills – from students and residents to experienced surgeons across many medical specialties. Surgery is first learned visually. Often, we see before and after photographs and wonder what took place in between. Our goal is to provide step-by-step instructions through a series of detailed color photographs illustrating the technique in between.

The field of dermatologic surgery has advanced tremendously over the last few decades. Once limited to relatively simple repairs, dermatologic surgery now encompasses major reconstructive surgical techniques. This atlas is a culmination of the years of experience gained by the authors in the surgical management of skin cancers. The defects are from a variety of locations, although mainly centered on the head and neck. The repairs vary in type and size in order to provide multiple reconstructive options. The photographs do not necessarily represent the best outcomes but are the highest-quality photographs that illustrate the full steps involved in the reconstruction. We believe that there are many ways to repair a defect, and the surgeon must understand all the different possibilities and ultimately be flexible in order to yield the best results. As such, we have provided as many variations as possible. The atlas can be studied in depth or used as a quick reference during surgery; its visual nature allows for both.

Although the authors are dermatologic surgeons, our experiences stem from the cooperation and shared learning with our surgical colleagues in head and neck oncology, surgical oncology, plastic surgery, oculoplastic surgery, and facial plastic surgery.

Acknowledgment

This atlas could not have been written without the help and support of many individuals. First and foremost, I would like thank the nursing and administrative staff for helping in the care of these patients and assisting me to collect the many photographs needed for this atlas. Heather Jones, Kitty Ware, David Schlicting, Melita Sheets, Justin Webb, Robyn Vazquez, Maria Samaan, Skye Fraser, Elizabeth Huff, and Ellen De Young – your help was invaluable. Many Fellows and residents contributed in the care as well. Thanks to the dermatologic surgery Fellows – Khosrow Mark Mehrany, Weimin Hu, Valencia Thomas, and Andrea Willey.

I would like to thank my coauthors Neil Swanson and Han Lee – Neil for his mentorship throughout my career and Han for encouraging me to write this atlas.

Finally, special thanks to my family for their loving support – my parents (Byung-Moon and Suzy), wife (Sonia), and children (Jessica and Stephen).

Ken Lee

CHAPTER 1

SUTURING TECHNIQUES

One of the cornerstones of cutaneous surgery is suturing. Mastering the various suturing techniques is paramount to achieving both a good aesthetic and functional outcome.

In order to obtain this goal one must understand the principles behind suturing. Without proper suturing, even the best planned reconstructions may not yield the best results.

The best scars result from wounds that are closed under minimal tension with good eversion of the wound edges. This is best achieved through layered suturing – placement of buried sutures followed by superficial cutaneous sutures.

This chapter illustrates the various suturing techniques used to obtain these results.

References

1. Adams B, Anwar J, Wrone DA, Alam M: Techniques for cutaneous sutured closures: variants and indications. Semin Cutan Med Surg 2003 Dec; 22(4): 306–16.
2. Zitelli JA, Moy RL. Buried vertical mattress suture. J Dermatol Surg Oncol 1989; 15: 17–9.
3. Swanson NA. Atlas of Cutaneous Surgery. Boston, MA: Little, Brown and Company. 1987.

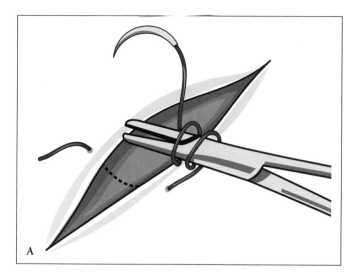

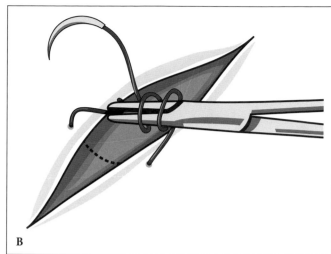

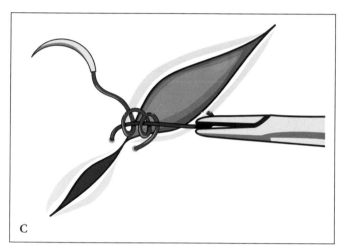

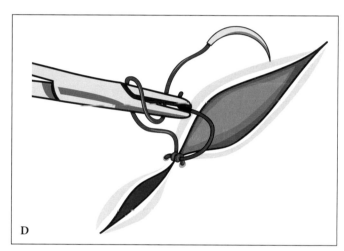

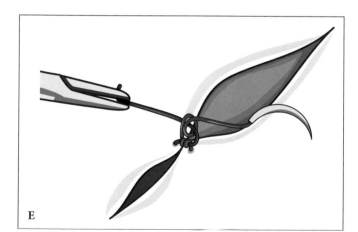

Figure 1.1 Square Knot. It is essential to master the square knot, which is used to secure the sutures. The square knot can be performed easily with a needle holder.

A. The first throw of the square knot requires looping the long end of the suture twice around the needle holder. **B.** Grasp the short end of the suture. **C.** Pull the needle holder through to the side where the needle exited. **D.** The second throw is made by looping the suture in the opposite direction once around the needle holder. **E.** Grasp the short end of the suture and pull the needle holder in the opposite direction of first throw. This is an important step to achieve a more secure square knot versus a granny knot. Repeat the sequence looping and pulling in opposite directions with each throw. Three to four throws are needed.

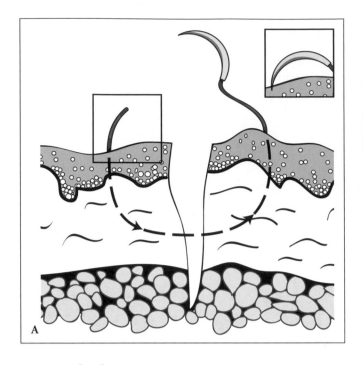
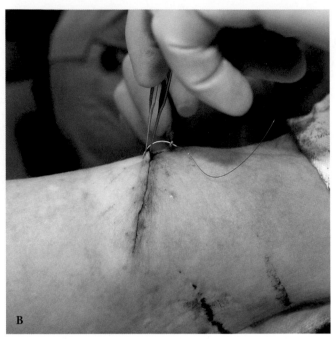
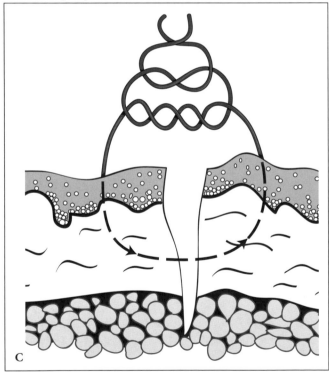
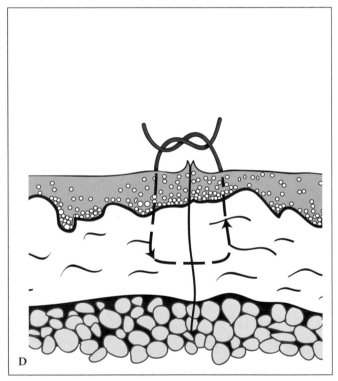

Figure 1.2 Simple Interrupted Suture. The simple interrupted stitch is the fundamental stitch used in dermatologic surgery.

A. Proper insertion of the needle point is a key component of achieving an optimal stitch. Begin with the needle point perpendicular to the skin surface or even pointing slightly outward, then allow the natural curved shape of the needle to follow through to the center and then to the other side of the wound edge in a flask-shaped path. **B.** Gently lifting the skin edge can ease the outward flare. **C.** Suture follows a flask-shaped path. **D.** This creates eversion of the wound edges.

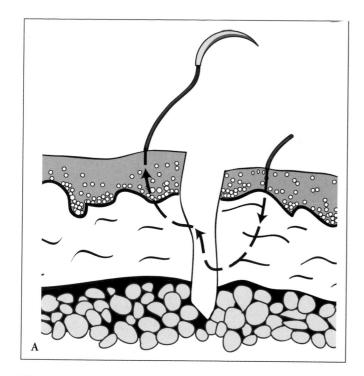
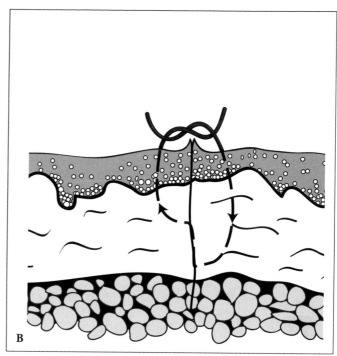

Figure 1.3 Correcting Uneven Wound Heights. The simple interrupted suture can also be used to adjust wounds of uneven heights by varying the depth of suture placement on either side of the wound.

A. The needle enters the low side more deeply and the high side more superficially. **B.** Level wound heights.

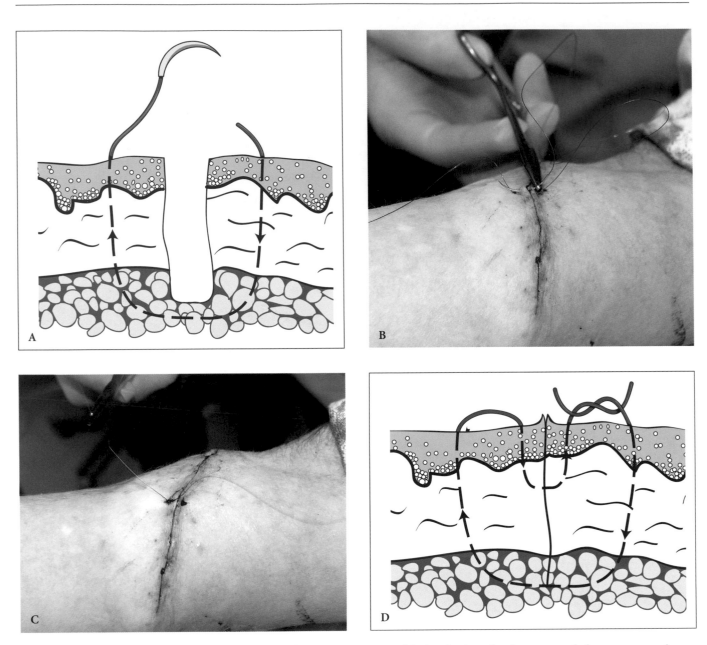

Figure 1.4 Vertical Mattress Suture. Vertical mattress suture aids in closing dead space and decreases tension while providing controlled wound eversion.

A. The first pass starts further from the wound edge, the starting point of which is determined by the amount of tension on the wound; the greater the tension, the deeper and wider the stitch, with both sides of the wound equidistant from the wound edges. **B.** The second pass starts in the opposite direction of the first pass and is a shorter and shallower stitch, but also of equal distance from the wound edges to provide even eversion. **C, D.** The suture is tied in the same technique as the simple interrupted suture.

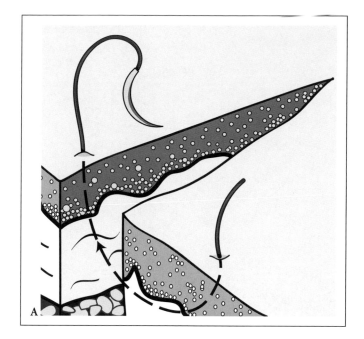

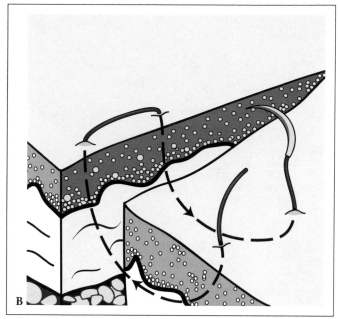

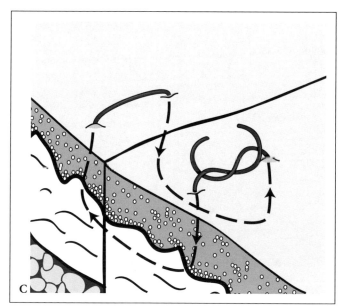

Figure 1.5 Horizontal Mattress. Horizontal mattress stitch is used to reduce tension and evert the wound edges.

A. Initially, the needle is passed through the skin similar to the simple interrupted suture. The needle is then reversed and passed through on the same side a few millimeters down from the exit point of the first pass. **B.** The needle then exits on the opposite side where the suture originated. **C.** Tied off with a square knot.

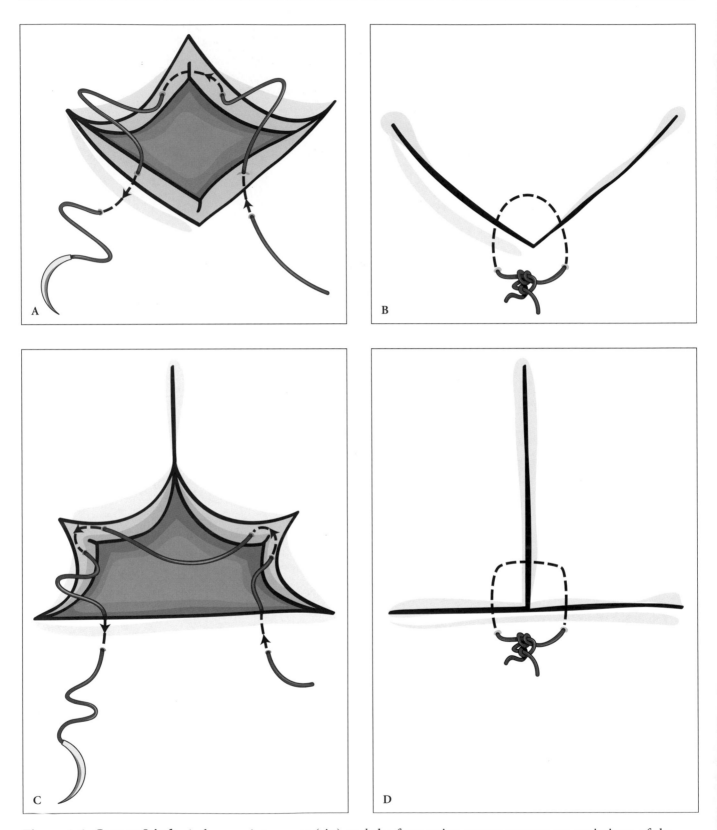

Figure 1.6 Corner Stitch. A three-point corner (tip) and the four-point corner sutures are variations of the horizontal mattress suture. These sutures are used to secure the corners in flaps.

A. Make the initial pass through the non-flap side of the incision. Pass the needle horizontally through the dermis of the flap. Enter the opposite side of the incision at the same level of the dermis and then exiting the skin. **B.** The tip is secured with a square knot. **C, D.** Four-point variation.

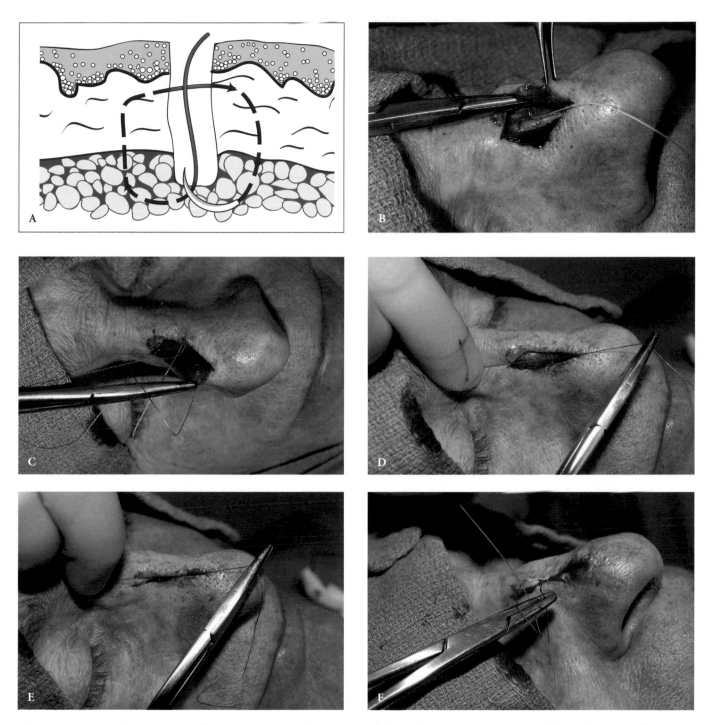

Figure 1.7 Buried Interrupted Suture. Proper placement of the subcutaneous or dermal buried suture allows for maximal wound eversion and decreases tension across the wound.

A. Simple variation. Begin with the needle in the deep dermis or fat and exit more superficially in the dermis. Enter the opposite side of the wound at the same depth and exit the needle deep in the wound and bring the needle out of the skin through the center. **B.** Needle path entering the undersurface of the dermis and exiting out of the superficial dermis. **C.** Needle then passes from superficial dermis to the undersurface of the dermis. **D, E.** The suture is tied in a square knot after the initial double loop similar to the cutaneous simple interrupted. However, the needle holder is pulled parallel to the wound. **F.** A second single loop is thrown in the opposite direction and the tail end grasped.

(Continued on next page.)

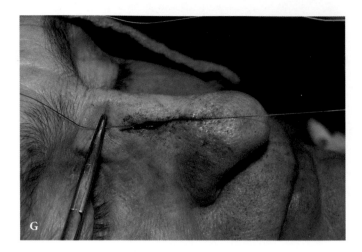
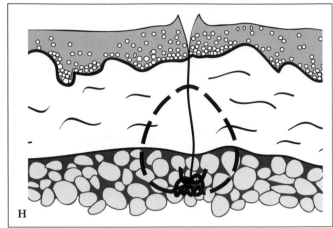
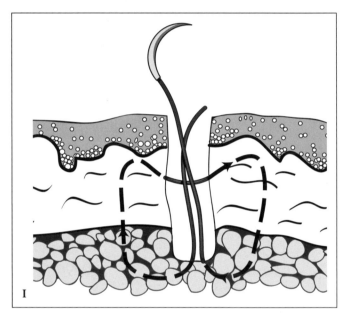
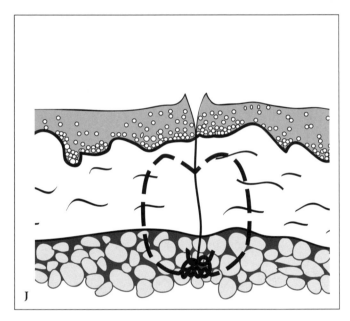

Figure 1.7 Buried Interrupted Suture *(continued).*

G. Needle holder is pulled in the opposite direction from the Figure 1.7D. **H.** The suture is cut on the knot usually after three ties and is buried deep in the tissue which results in less suture-spitting on the surface of the wound. **I, J.** Vertical Mattress Variation. For even greater wound eversion, the needle is pointed upward, toward the epidermis, in order to create a heart-shaped path. The dermis needs to be thick enough to allow for this.

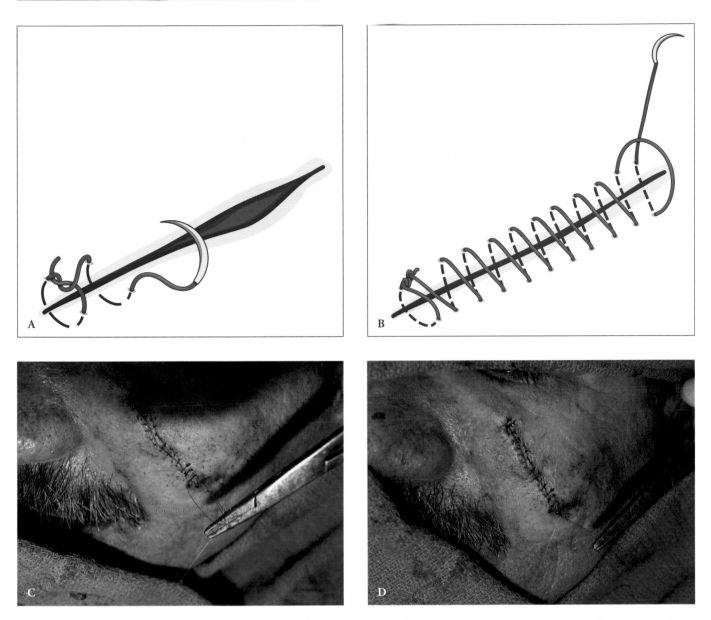

Figure 1.8 Running Cutaneous Sutures. When wounds are under minimal tension, continuously running the cutaneous suture can save time.

A. Simple Running Suture Variation. Simple interrupted suture is tied but only the short end is cut. The longer needle end is continuously passed through the skin in series. **B.** At the end, a short loop is brought out from the final pass. **C, D.** The longer needle end of the suture is then tied off with the loop that serves as the tail end.

(Continued on next page.)

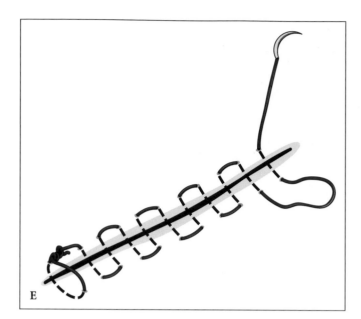
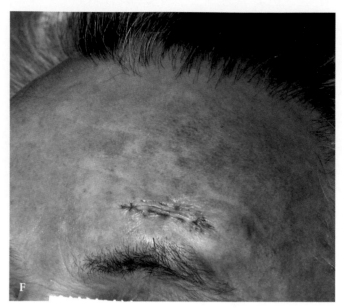

Figure 1.8 Running Cutaneous Sutures *(continued).*

E. Running Horizontal Mattress Variation. Started in the same way as the standard horizontal mattress suture, but the needle is continuously looped in a series of horizontal mattress sutures. At the end, the suture is tied onto itself by creating a loop with the final pass. **F.** This technique produces tremendous eversion and is particularly useful in creases to prevent indentation.

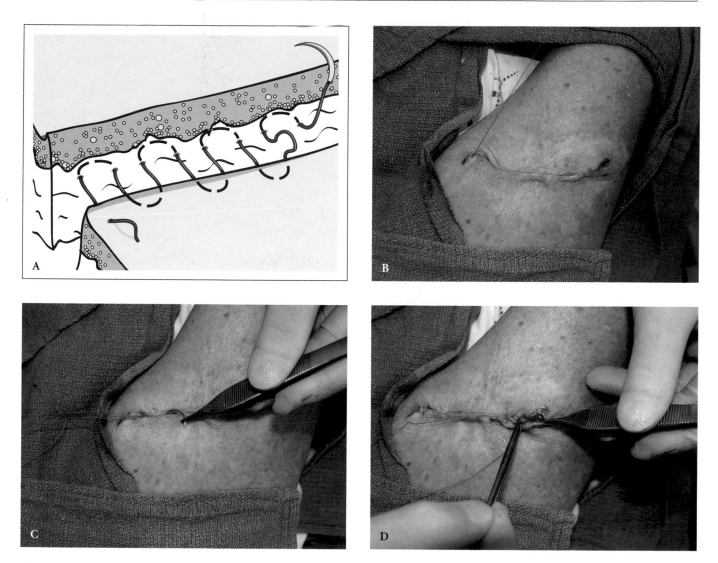

Figure 1.9 Running Subcuticular Sutures.

A. The running subcuticular stitch prevents unwanted track marks on the skin surface and can be performed with either absorbable or nonabsorbable suture. When using absorbable suture, the starting end is a simple buried suture but only the tail end is cut. The needle snakes back and forth in the upper dermis. At the end, the suture is tied onto itself by creating a loop with the final pass. **B.** Buried dermal suture with tail end cut. **C.** Horizontal pass through the upper dermis. **D.** Needle through the dermis on the opposite side after several back and forth weaves.

(Continued on next page.)

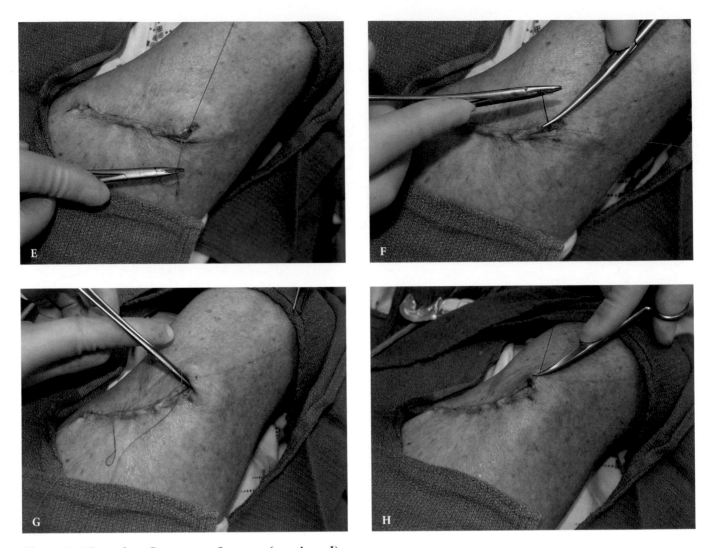

Figure 1.9 Running Cutaneous Sutures *(continued).*

E. Loop made from the final pass. **F.** Knot tied then only the tail end is cut at the knot. **G.** The needle is passed through the end of the incision and exited through the skin pulling the knot deeper. **H.** The remaining suture is cut at the level of the skin thereby leaving no remnants of the suture.

CHAPTER 2

SIMPLE EXCISION AND REPAIR

The fusiform ellipse is a fundamental excisional technique in cutaneous surgery. Mastering this technique along with its variations lays the groundwork for the successful development of more complicated techniques.

As a general rule, the ideal length-to-width ratio of a fusiform elliptical excision is 3 to 1; this maximizes the probability of achieving the ideal angle at the apices of the ellipse of 30°. However, the ratio can vary depending on the inherent characteristics of the skin in various anatomic locations, as well as the elasticity of the skin. The incorporation of the ideal ratio and ideal angle of the fusiform ellipse enables the repair to be performed without leaving an undesired pucker of redundant skin, also called a dog-ear, at either end of the closure.

The fusiform ellipse is usually placed along the relaxed skin tension lines (RSTL). Repairs designed along RSTL reduces the tension on the wound edge, resulting in a better scar.

Variations of the fusiform ellipse include the curved ellipse, "lazy-S" excision, and M-plasty. These surgical techniques take into consideration that RSTL do not always fit neatly into straight lines and allow for customization of the scar to anatomic regions.

References

1.   Borges AF. Relaxed skin tension lines (RSTL) versus other skin lines. Plast Reconstr Surg 1984; 73:144.
2.   Swanson NA. Atlas of Cutaneous Surgery. Boston, MA: Little, Brown and Company. 1987.

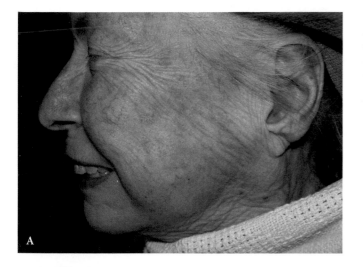

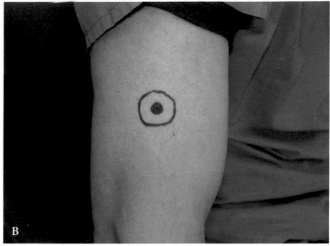

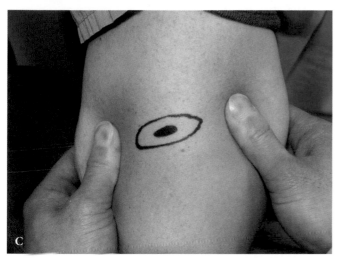

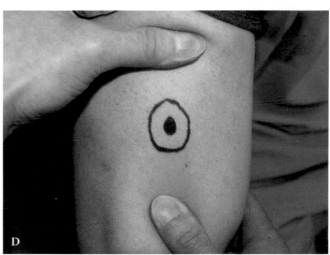

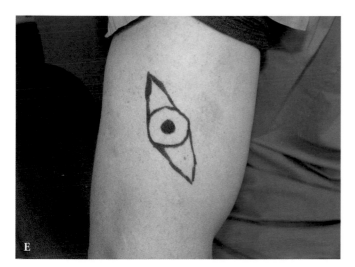

Figure 2.1 Relaxed Skin Tension Lines(RSTL).

A. In older individuals, the RSTL will be obvious as they coincide with wrinkles. However, in younger individuals these lines can be accentuated with exaggerated facial movements such as smiling, grimacing, and pursing the lips. This accentuates the RSTL of the face and helps one determine the direction of the fusiform ellipse. **B, C.** When performing surgery on the neck, trunk, and extremities, where lines and tension can change depending on the position, the RSTL is best determined by stretching the skin with the patient in a neutral position. The RSTL is perpendicular to the direction of maximum distensibility. **D.** Note that the skin is less distensible when stretched in the opposite direction. **E.** Fusiform ellipse drawn along the RSTL.

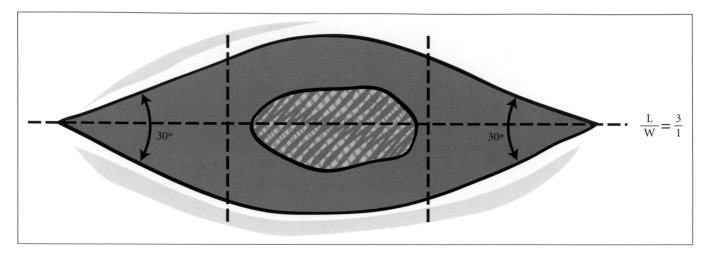

Figure 2.2 Fusiform Ellipse.

The ideal length-to-width ratio of an elliptical excision is 3 to 1 and the ideal angle is 30°. These proportions allow for the closure to be achieved with minimal to no redundant cones of tissue (dog-ears) on either end of the wound.

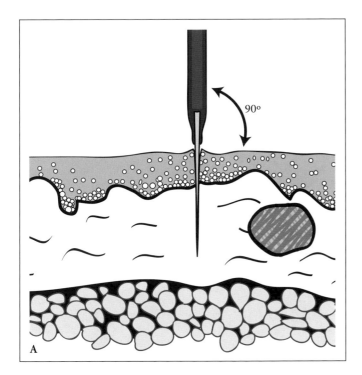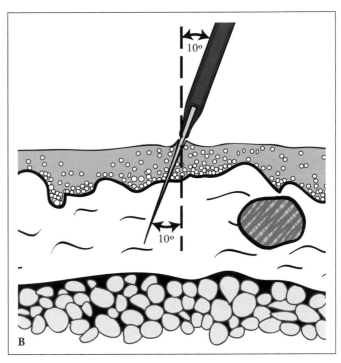

Figure 2.3 Scalpel Angle.

A. The scalpel should be upright and perpendicular to the skin while making the incision. **B.** In some instances, a slight bevel of the blade out will allow for closer reapproximation of the skin-wound edges.

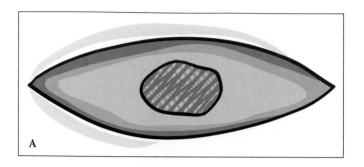

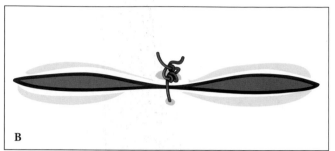

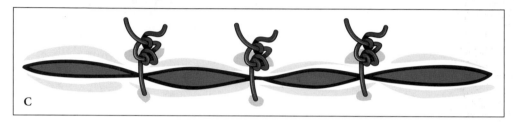

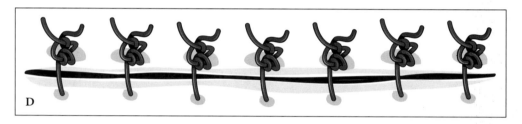

Figure 2.4 Rule of Halves.

A. The rule of halves in the repair of a simple ellipse allows for optimal alignment of the wound edge and the tension to be distributed evenly throughout the wound length. **B.** The first suture is placed in the middle of the wound. **C.** Subsequent sutures are placed by bisecting each half in sequential fashion.

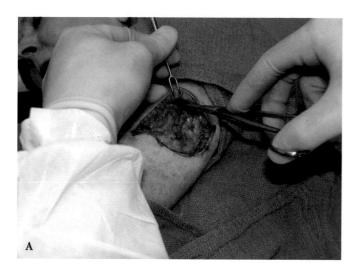
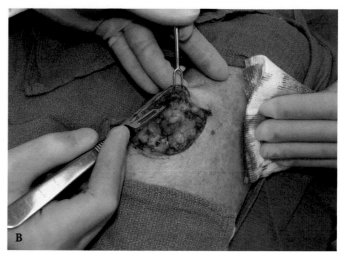

Figure 2.5 Undermining. Undermining can be performed either by blunt or sharp dissection.

A. Blunt dissection using scissors to spread the fat. This is the safer method and preferable for less experienced surgeons. **B.** Sharp dissection is faster but is more likely to lead to undermining in the wrong plane or injuring important structures such as nerves and vessels. This should be reserved for more experienced surgeons.

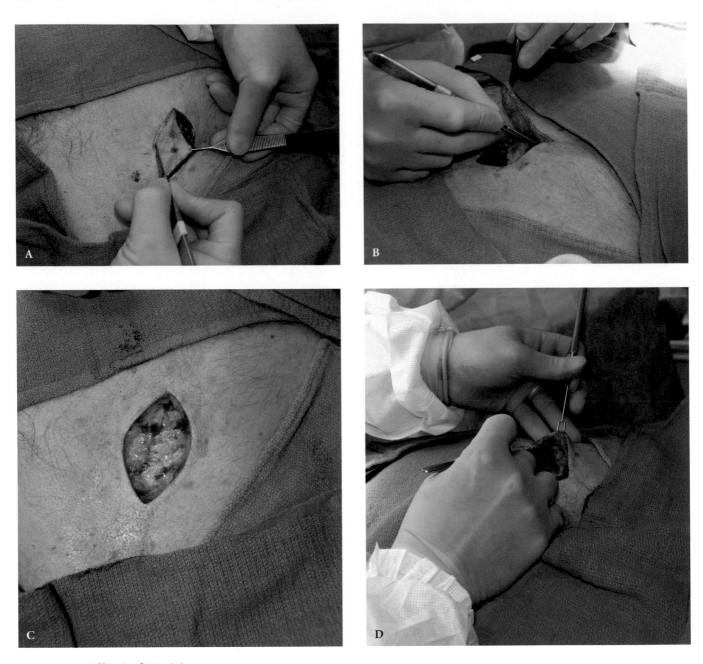

Figure 2.6 Elliptical Excision.

A. Once the ellipse is designed, it is excised with the blade beveled slightly outward. Countertraction makes the skin taut and facilitates the incision. **B.** The tissue is removed at a consistent depth of the tissue plane so that the same amount of fat is left at the base. **C.** Defect resulting from removal of an ellipse. Note the sharp vertical skin edges and the flat base of the wound. **D.** Wound edges are undermined in all directions to decrease tension and to optimize wound-edge eversion. **E.** In this layered closure, the fascia is closed first to further decrease tension. **F.** The dermis is closed applying the rule of halves. **G.** The surface layer is closed with absorbable running subcuticular sutures. Note the excellent wound eversion. **H.** Two years post-op: the scar has spread minimally due to the design along RSTL.

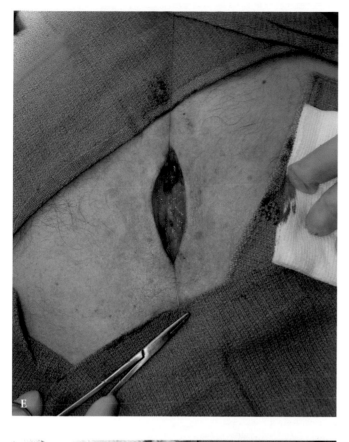

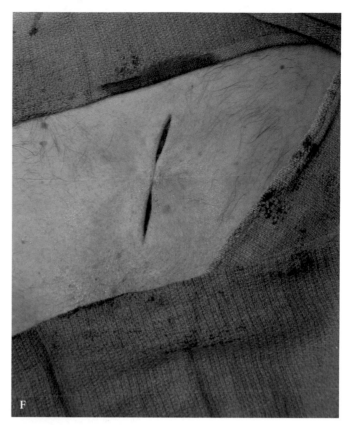

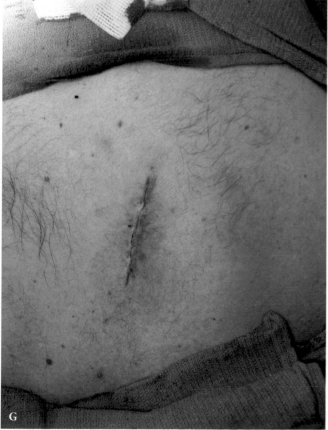

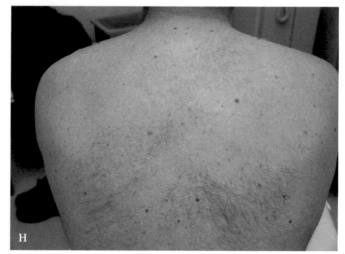

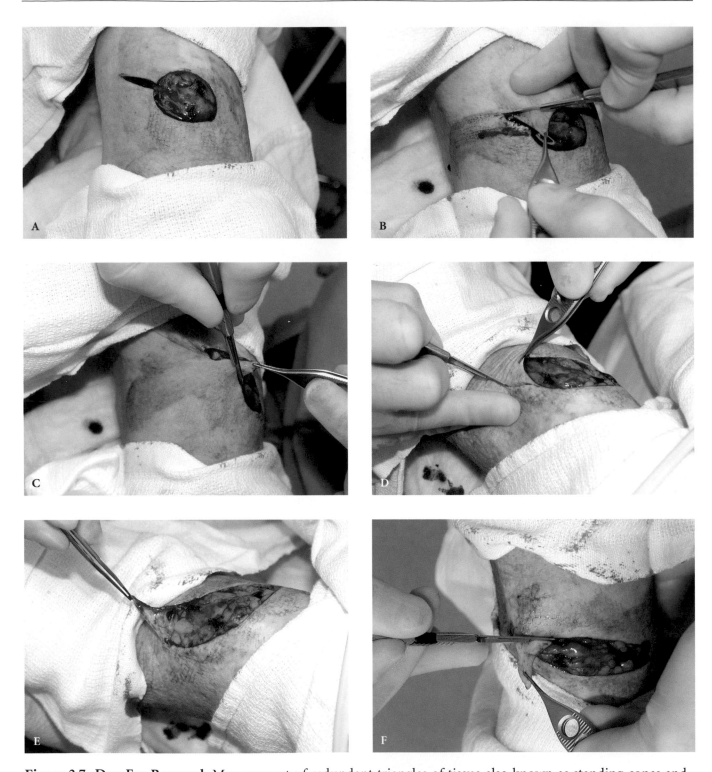

Figure 2.7 Dog-Ear Removal. Management of redundant triangles of tissue also known as standing cones and dog-ears is important as the fusiform ellipse does not always fit perfectly as designed and excess skin remains. There are two methods.

A. One technique involves removing two smaller triangles of tissue; an incision is made extending from the center of the defect to the furthest point of the excess tent of tissue. **B, C.** The two triangles are then excised on each side and tapered to blend with the defect. **D.** The other method involves making an incision along the desired final suture line; this line extends to the end of the excess tissue. **E, F.** The resulting triangle of tissue is undermined and draped over the suture line and excised. This technique has the advantage of only needing two incisions.

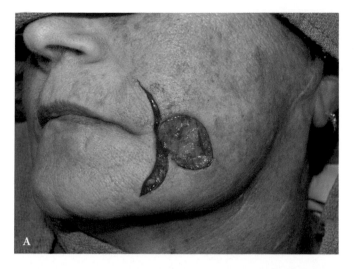

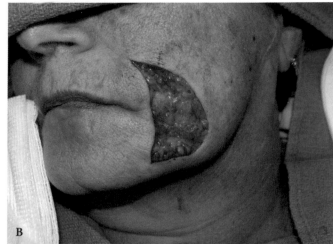

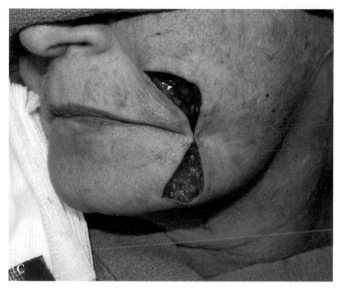

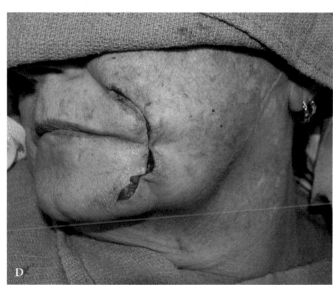

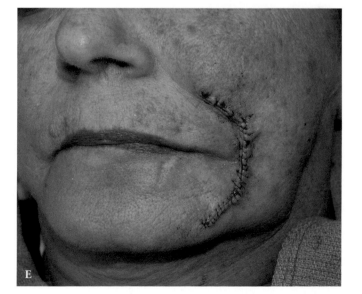

Figure 2.8 Curved Ellipse. A curved ellipse is created by closing wounds of unequal lengths.

A. The incision to create the inner aspect of the curve is shorter and straighter. **B.** The outer incision is longer and curved. **C.** The wound is then closed by the rule of halves with the key stitch in the middle of the wound. **D.** Further bisection of each half in sequential fashion helps distribute the tension and length evenly throughout the length of the wound. **E.** The curved ellipse is particularly useful to camouflage scars within naturally occurring curves such as the melolabial fold.

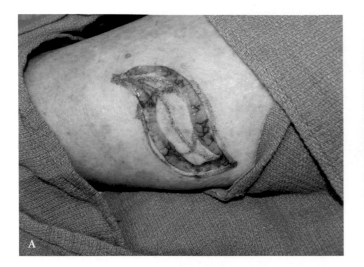

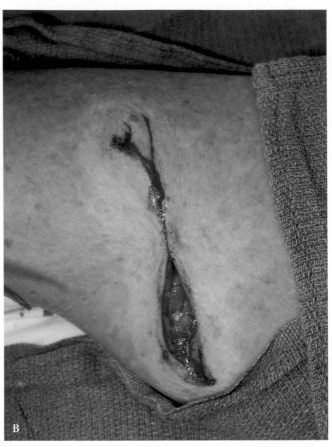

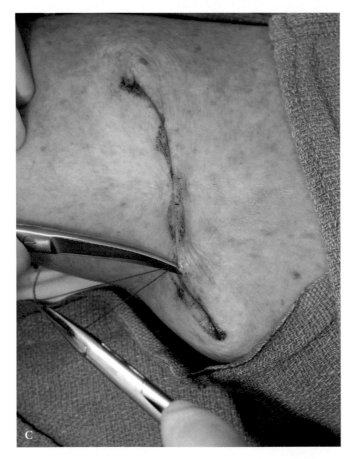

Figure 2.9 Lazy-S. A "lazy-S" ellipse creates two curves in opposite directions. It helps taper the excessive puckering that can occur on convexities such as the extremities.

A. The excision is designed in a "lazy-S" shape. **B, C.** The wound is then closed by the rule of halves with the key stitch in the middle of the wound. Further bisection of each half in sequential fashion results in an "S" shape.

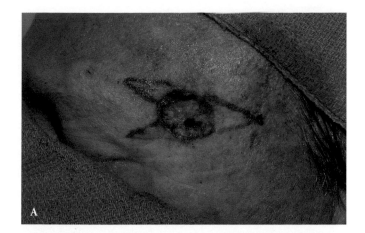

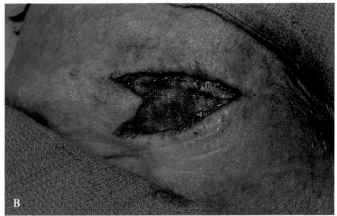

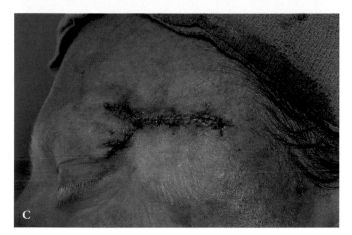

Figure 2.10 M-plasty. An M-plasty is used to prevent the extension of an incision into significant cosmetic areas such as the eyebrows. The M-plasty is used to wrap the incisions above and below the eyebrow.

A. The design of the M-plasty involves creating two 30° angles at one end of the fusiform ellipse; this shortens the length of the scar by one-fourth to one-third. **B.** Three tips are excised. **C.** Immediate post-op. A three-point tip stitch is useful at the corner of the M-plasty.

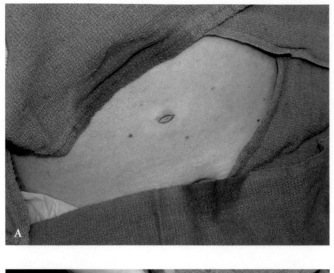

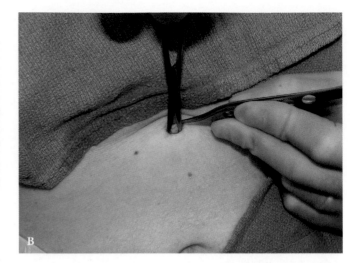

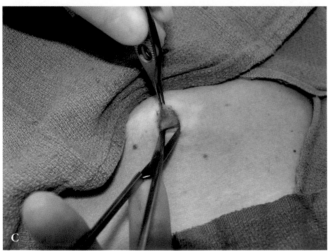

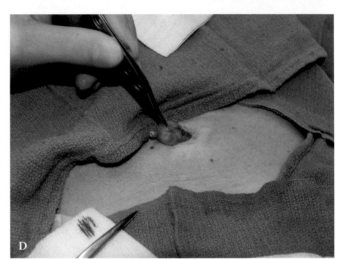

Figure 2.11 Cyst Excision. The goal of cyst surgery is to remove the cyst intact through an incision that is smaller than the cyst.

A. A narrow incisional fusiform ellipse is made around the cyst punctum. **B.** Forceps are used grasp the elliptical piece of skin to provide upward traction in order to facilitate the identification of the plane around the cyst sac. **C.** Dissection is continued underneath the cyst in order to free it from the surrounding tissue. **D.** Cyst is removed intact. **E.** Small incision sutured closed.

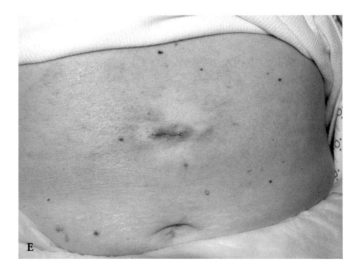

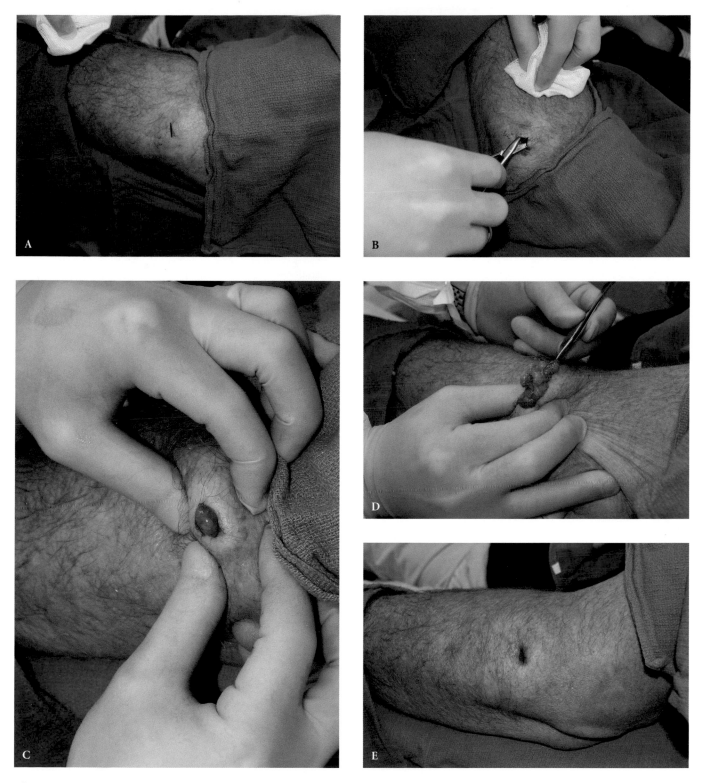

Figure 2.12 Lipoma Excision. The goal of lipoma removal is similar to cyst surgery but through even a smaller incision.

A. Small stab incision made through the center of the skin overlying the lipoma. **B.** Blunt dissection is performed around the entire lipoma. Unlike a cyst, there is no lining. **C.** With very firm pressure, the lipoma is expressed. **D.** As more of the lipoma is expressed out, forceps can be used to provide gentle traction. **E.** After complete removal.

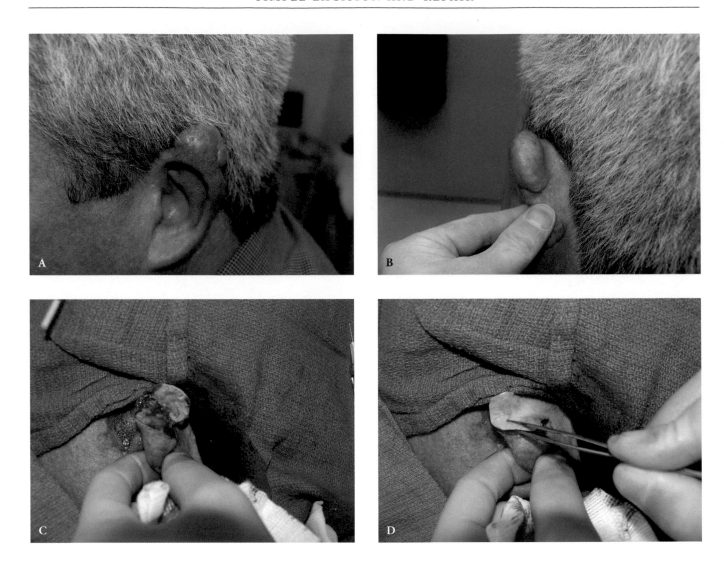

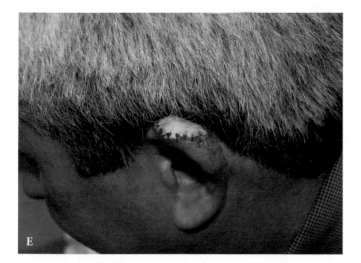

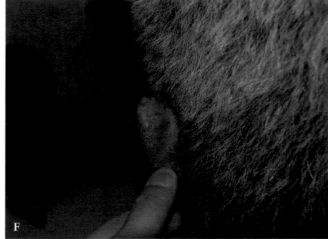

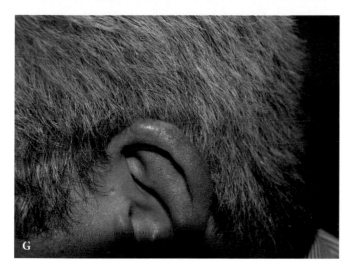

Figure 2.13 Keloid Excision. Keloids have a tendency to recur. Excision should be accompanied by intralesional steroids and pressure.

A, B. Keloid on upper ear helix. **C.** Incision made around the base of the keloid leaving it attached posteriorly. The keloid is "shelled out" and excess skin is trimmed. **D.** The trimmed keloid skin is laid down with no tension. **E.** Immediate post-op. **F, G.** Five-month post-op after serial intralesional steroid injections.

CHAPTER 3

OVERVIEW OF FLAPS

A *flap* is defined as the movement of adjacent skin and subcutaneous tissue with its vascular supply intact. Flaps are classified according to location, blood supply, and movement. This atlas will focus on flaps that arise from adjacent or near adjacent tissue. These flaps derive their blood supply either from a random pattern or an axial pattern (based on a named artery).

Before performing flap surgery, a thorough understanding of flap nomenclature, principles, and dynamics is required.

1. The primary defect is the original wound to be closed.
2. The secondary defect is the wound created by the movement of flap in order to close the primary defect.
3. The primary motion of the flap is the motion or stress placed on it to close the primary defect.
4. The secondary motion is the motion or stress placed on the tissue surrounding the primary defect by the flap.

Therefore, there is a combination of primary and secondary wounds and primary and secondary motions for every flap design and execution. Understanding the direction of the resulting vector forces is critical.

A classic description of flaps is based on their movement: advancement, rotation, and transposition. Advancement flaps are the simplest of the flaps to conceptualize and entail the movement of the adjacent tissue along a single vector. Rotation flaps rotate around a single pivot point along a radiating arc. Transposition flaps are flaps that are lifted and transposed over intervening skin.

Flap movement can also be divided into two categories: sliding and lifting. Sliding encompasses rotating and/or advancing adjacent tissue into a defect. It is unusual to have just a pure rotation or advancement; therefore, sliding may be an easier way to understand tissue movement.

Table 3.1 Flap Classification

Sliding Flaps	Lifting Flaps
Advancement	Transposition
Rotation	Bilobe
Island Pedicle	Rhombic
	Interpolated

Lifting flaps encompass movement of the flap over intervening skin. This could be either transposing adjacent skin or interpolating near adjacent skin. (Table 3.1). This classification also allows for the addition of other specialized flaps, like the island pedicle and interpolated flap.

This chapter illustrates the design, principle, and basic application of the common flaps.

More specific applications and the long-term results will be covered in the subsequent chapters.

References

1. Bray DA. Rhombic Flaps. In: Baker SR, Swanson NA. Local Flaps in Facial Reconstruction. St. Louis: Mosby, Inc.; 1995. p. 151–64.
2. Dzubow LM. Advancement Flaps. In: Dzubow LM. Facial Flaps Biomechanics and Regional Application. Norwalk: Appleton & Lange; 1990. p. 22–30.
3. Papadopoulos DJ, Trinei FA. Superiorly based nasalis myocutaneous island pedicle flap with bilevel undermining for nasal tip and supratip reconstruction. Dermatol Surg 1999 Jul; 25(7): 530–6.
4. Vecchione TR, Griffith L. Closure of scalp defects by using multiple flaps in a pinwheel design. Plast Reconstr Surg 1978; 62: 74–80.
5. Webster RC, Davidson TM, Smith RC: The thirty-degree transposition flap. Laryngoscope 88(1 Pt 1): 85–94, 1978.
6. Zitelli JA, The bilobed flap for nasal reconstruction. Arch Dermatol 125(7): 957–9, 1989.

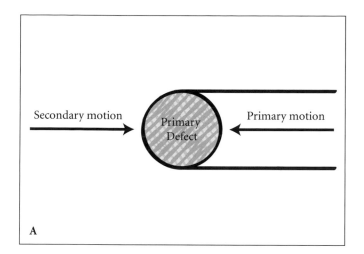

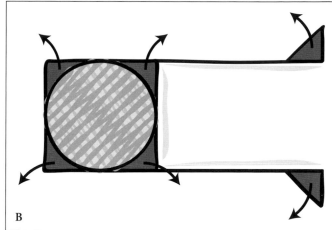

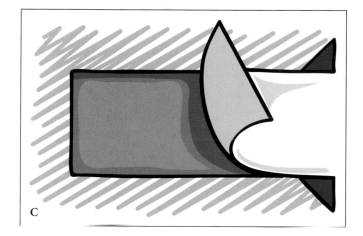

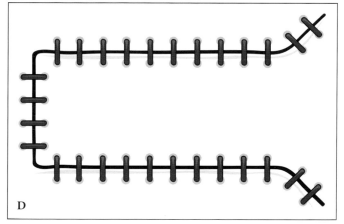

Figure 3.1 Advancement Flap.

A. The single advancement is a useful flap in certain anatomic sites such as the eyebrow and forehead. The flap relies on the elasticity of the skin and has a relatively narrow blood supply compared to other advancement flaps. Therefore, the flap must be designed so that the base does not become narrow. **B.** The circular defect is trimmed to convert it into a square. Burow's triangles can be removed anywhere along the incision, but are often removed at the base of the flap. **C.** The flap is elevated and undermined in the shaded regions. **D.** Note the slight widening of the flap base.

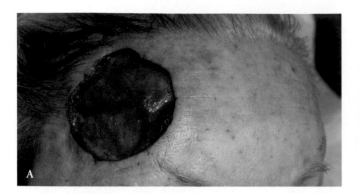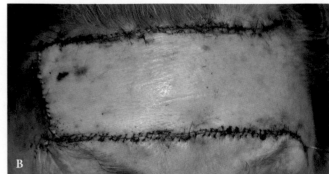

Figure 3.2 Advancement Flap.

A. The forehead is an ideal location for the classic advancement flap, as the incisions are parallel to the forehead creases. **B.** Immediate post-op. A second flap can be designed on the opposite side for a bilateral advancement flap, sometimes called an H-plasty. Note the slight widening of the flap base located on the right of the photo. This ensures that the vascular pedicle is not compromised.

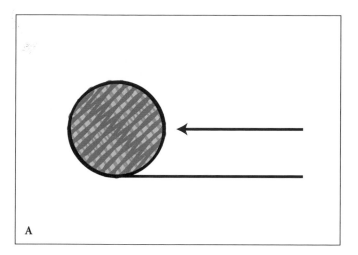

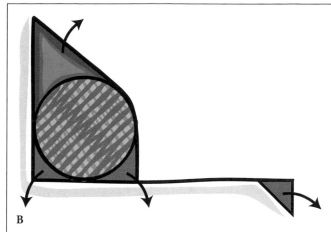

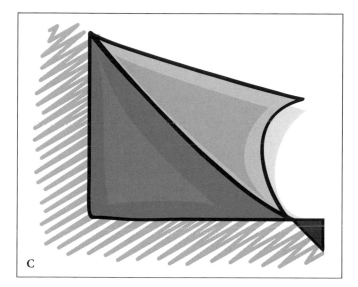

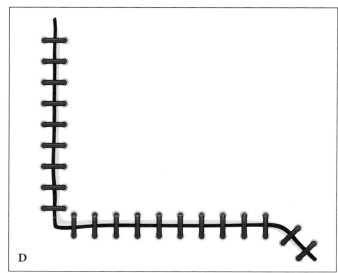

Figure 3.3 Advancement Flap.

A. The advancement flap has many variations. "O to L" or "A to L" is a common variation. A single horizontal incision is made at the base of the defect, usually along a cosmetic border. **B.** A dog-ear is removed in a direction perpendicular to the original incision. **C.** The flap is elevated and undermined in the shaded regions. **D.** Because the incisions are perpendicular, there is a wide vascular pedicle at the base of the flap. An additional horizontal incision in the opposite direction would provide more movement and is called an "O to T" or "A to T" advancement flap.

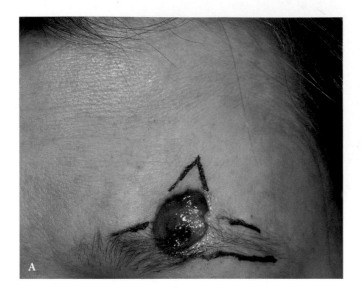 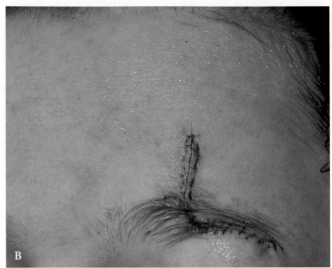

Figure 3.4 Advancement Flap.

A. An "O to L" flap is chosen due to the anatomic constraints of the region. A single advancement flap following the contours of the eyebrow would result in a narrow base. **B.** Immediate post-op. Note that the horizontal incision is made along the inferior cosmetic border of the eyebrow. It is important that the flap is undermined at a level below the hair follicles so as not to damage them.

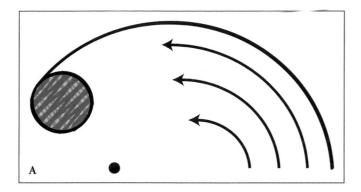

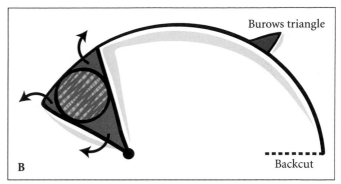

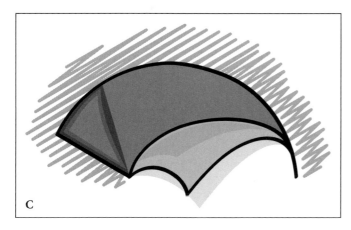

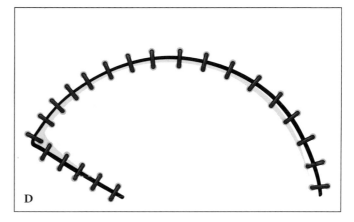

Figure 3.5 Rotation Flap.

A. The rotation flap is designed with a long radiating arc incision. The flap rotates around a pivot point, and the movement is limited by the elasticity and mobility of the flap skin. **B.** Dog-ears are removed to essentially make the defect into a triangle with the inferior aspect of the triangle serving as the pivot point. A Burow's triangle can be removed anywhere along the length of the arc, or the incision can be made long enough in order to blend it out along the length. A back-cut made into the base of the flap can also be used if the base is wide enough. **C.** The flap is elevated and widely undermined in the shaded areas. **D.** The flap is draped into place. Rotation flaps can be performed with multiple incisions in areas like the scalp, where elasticity and mobility are limited.

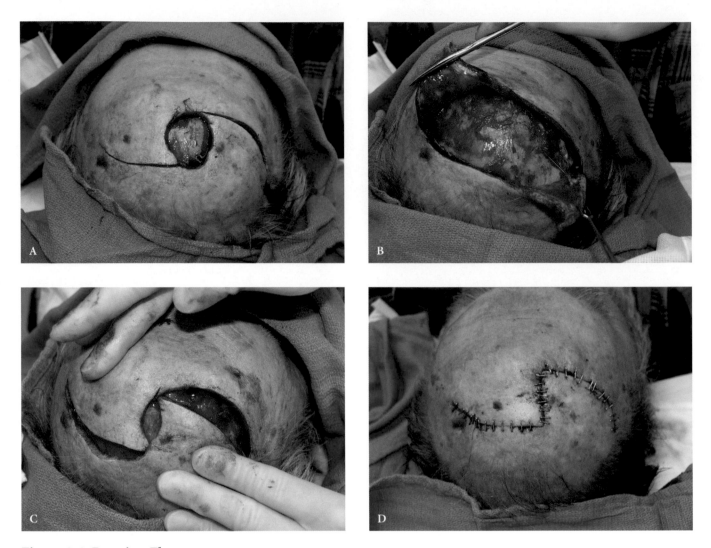

Figure 3.6 Rotation Flap.

A. Defect on the scalp. Two long arcing incisions to create two rotation flaps. **B.** The flaps are undermined and lifted. **C.** Flaps are rotated into place. **D.** Immediate post-op.

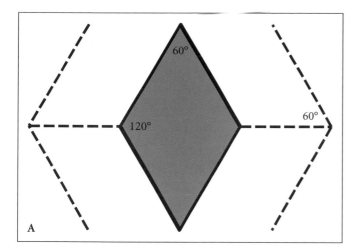

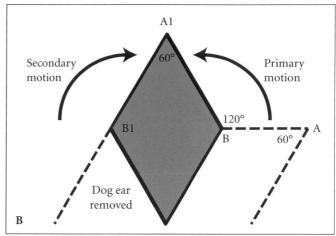

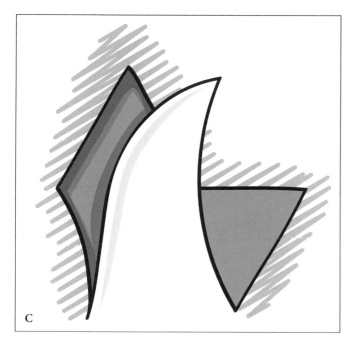

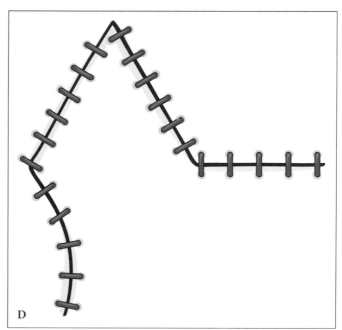

Figure 3.7 Rhombic Flap.

A. The classic rhombic transposition flap has four possible directions from which the flap can originate. **B.** The 60° triangular flap is matched to the 60° triangular defect tip. The flap travels 120° over intervening skin. The greater this angle, the larger the resulting dog-ear. **C.** The flap is elevated and widely undermined in the shaded areas. Unlike sliding flaps, the secondary defect is closed first, which facilitates the draping of the flap into the primary defect. **D.** The final shape of the flap. Note that the dog-ear was flared out so that the flap base is not compromised.

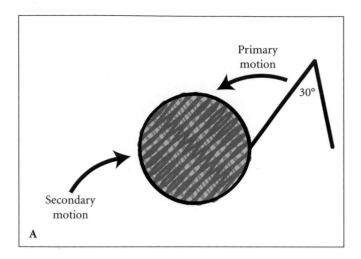

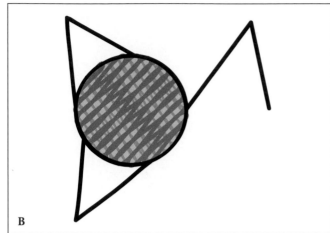

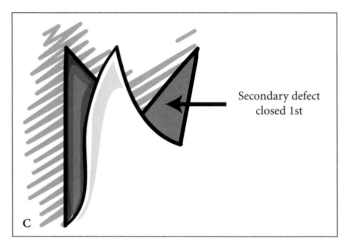

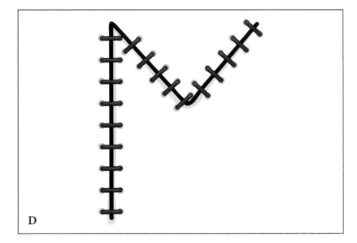

Figure 3.8 Rhombic Flap.

A. Webster and Dufourmental variations of the rhombic transposition flap applied to a circular defect. The flap is narrowed to 30° which makes the secondary defect easier to close but relies on a much greater secondary motion. The angle distance that the flap travels is smaller, leading to a smaller dog-ear. **B.** The defect is modified to accommodate the tip of the flap and the dog-ear is removed inferiorly. **C.** The flap is elevated and widely undermined in the shaded areas. The secondary defect is closed first, which facilitates the draping of the flap into the primary defect. **D.** The final shape of the flap. Note that the dog-ear removal was flared out so that the flap base is not compromised.

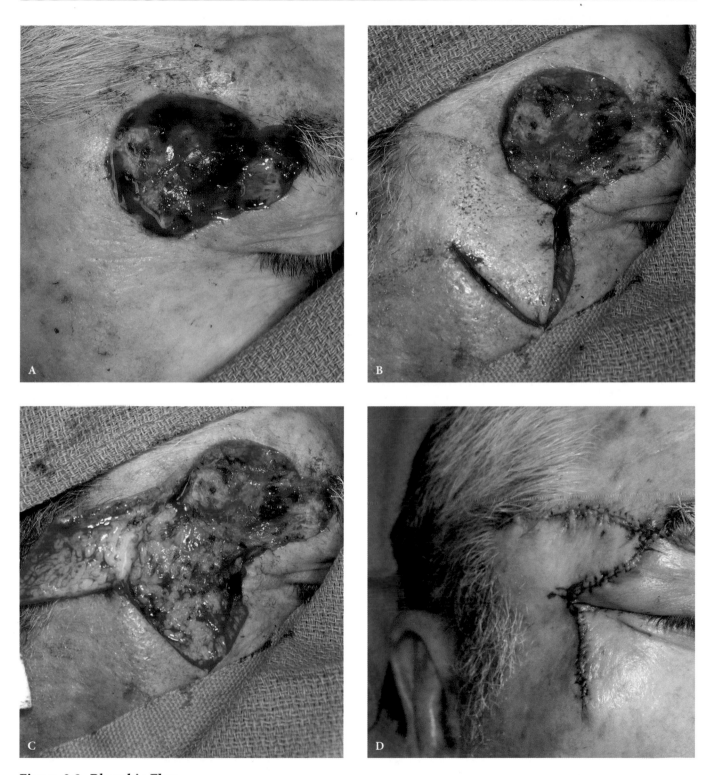

Figure 3.9 Rhombic Flap.

A. Complex defect involving the temple, eyebrow, and eyelid. The rhombic flap is particularly useful when there is no adjacent skin that can be easily slid into place. **B.** The skin inferior to the defect is chosen for the flap because of its elasticity and mobility. It is helpful to squeeze the skin around the perimeter of the defect in order to determine which location serves as the best source of the flap. **C.** The flap is elevated and the surrounding tissue undermined at the level of the subcutaneous fat. **D.** The flap is then draped into place, first closing the secondary defect and then securing the flap into the primary defect.

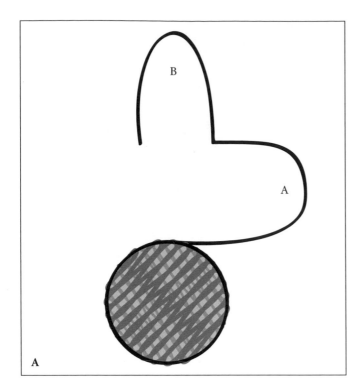

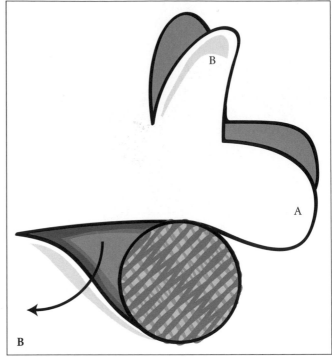

Figure 3.10 Bilobe Flap.

A. The classic bilobe flap is essentially a rhombic transposition flap done sequentially. The primary lobe A is transposed into the primary defect and the secondary lobe B transposed into the secondary defect. The tertiary defect is then closed primarily. The classic bilobe flap has 180° of movement. **B.** The flap is elevated, undermined widely in the shaded areas, and then transposed, which creates a dog-ear laterally. The dog-ear is relatively large because of the large angle distance traveled by the flap. **C.** The final shape of the flap. Note that the dog-ear removal was flared out so that the flap base is not compromised.

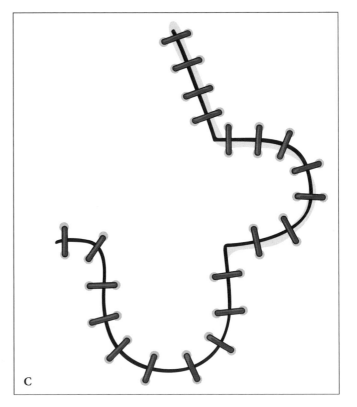

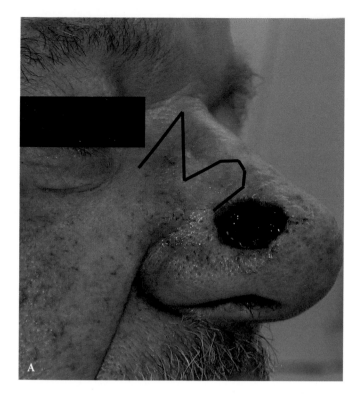

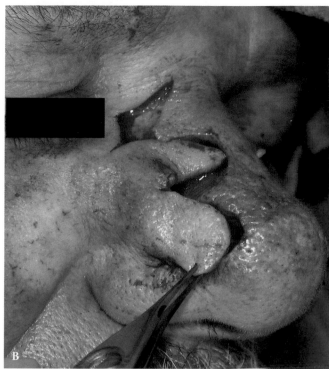

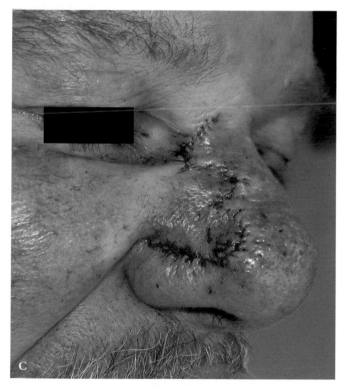

Figure 3.11 Bilobe Flap. Variation of the bilobe flap in which overall angle is approximately 90°.

A. Defect with bilobe incision outlined. The primary lobe is approximately the same size as the primary defect, and the secondary lobe is approximately 90% of the secondary defect. Undersizing these flaps will result in secondary motion elevating the nasal rim. **B.** The two lobes of the flap move into the defects in a stepwise fashion. **C.** The flap is draped and sutured into place with minimal dog-ear removal. Note the lack of distortion in the surrounding skin.

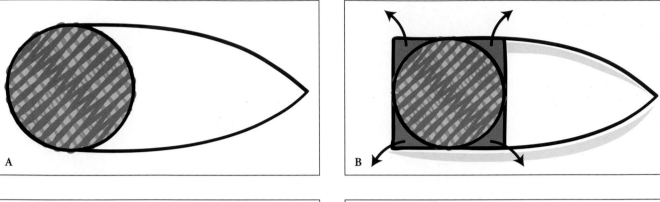

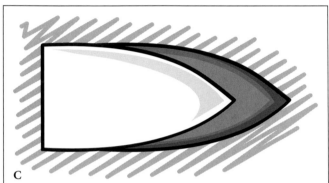

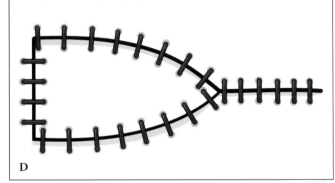

Figure 3.12 Island Pedicle Flap.

A. The island pedicle flap relies on a subcutaneous vascular pedicle located below the flap. The skin incision is made completely around the entire flap. The flap is undermined into the subcutaneous space and a small central pedicle is left. **B.** The flap is elevated and then advanced into the primary defect. The surrounding shaded area is widely undermined. **C.** The flap is freed from the surrounding tissue, leaving a small pedicle. **D.** The final shape of the flap. The island pedicle is sometimes called a "V to Y flap."

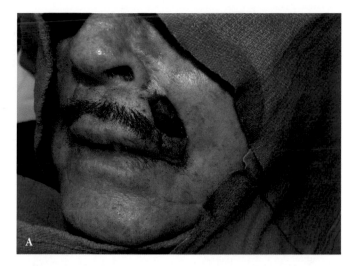

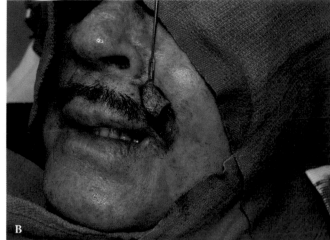

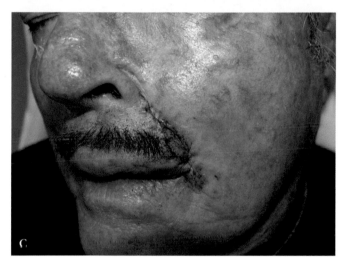

Figure 3.13 Island Pedicle Flap.

A. An island pedicle flap is designed from the inferior aspect with one incision line along the nasolabial fold. **B.** The flap is advanced into place attached by the subcutaneous pedicle. **C.** Immediate post-op. Note that the flap has been rotated as well as advanced and trimmed into an elliptical shape to better fit the contours of the anatomic region. The dog-ear was removed superiorly so that the superior border is tapered.

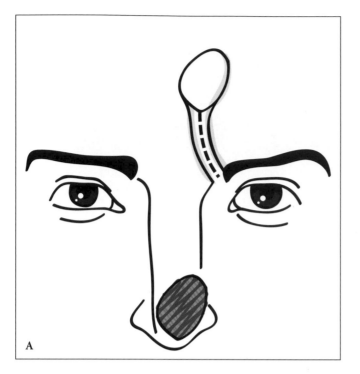

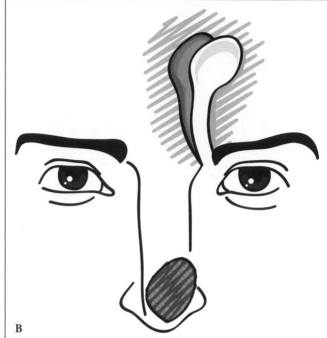

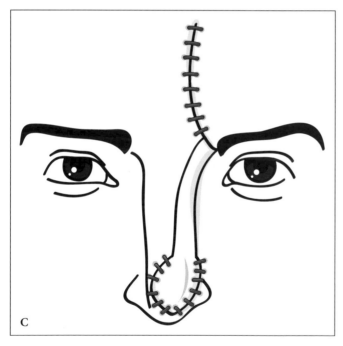

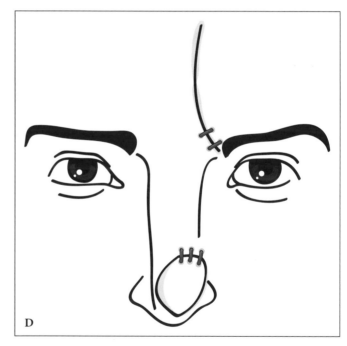

Figure 3.14 Interpolated Flap.

A. The paramedian forehead flap is a type of interpolated flap. An incision is made along the path of the supratrochlear artery and around a template of the defect. **B.** The flap is elevated and the shaded regions widely undermined. **C.** The pedicle base is interpolated and draped onto the primary defect. The defect on the forehead is closed primarily. **D.** The pedicle is detached 3 weeks later and the flap inset.

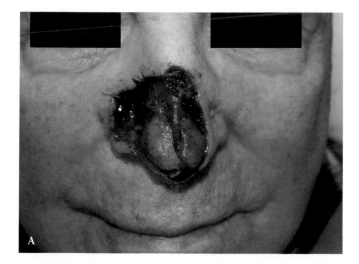

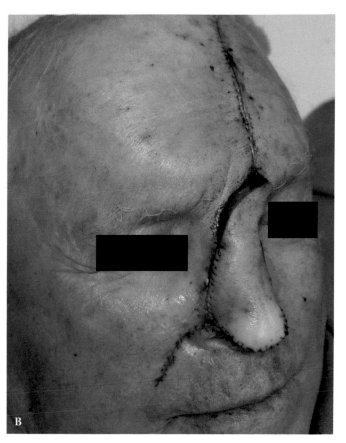

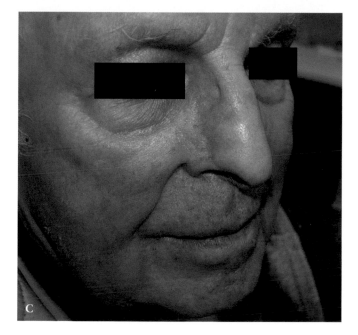

Figure 3.15 Interpolated Flap.

A. Defect involving the nasal tip, dorsum, sidewall, and ala. **B.** Immediate post-op. The paramedian forehead flap is interpolated and secured to the defect. The distal blanching is due to the epinephrine effect. The lateral portion of the defect closed with advancement flap. **C.** Post detachment. The pedicle is excised and the proximal and distal ends are set in.

CHAPTER 4

OVERVIEW OF GRAFTS

There are four main types of grafts used in cutaneous surgery: full-thickness skin graft, split-thickness skin graft, composite graft, and cartilage graft. All grafts are removed from the donor area, detached from the original blood supply, and then transferred to the recipient site where they must reform a new vascular attachment.

Full-thickness skin graft (FTSG) is comprised of the epidermis and the full complement of the dermis. The typical donor sites are conchal bowl, pre- and postauricular sulci for smaller defects, and clavicular and inguinal skin for larger defects. FTSG is used to achieve the best cosmetic match.

Split-thickness skin graft (STSG) is comprised of the epidermis and part of the dermis. STSG is typically used to cover larger defects where a FTSG would not be feasible. STSG varies in thickness to accommodate the defect. Additional equipment is needed to harvest the graft. Donor sites include posterior arms, thighs, lower abdomen, and buttocks where the resultant scar would be less conspicuous.

Composite graft is comprised of attached skin and cartilage. A composite graft is typically used in superficial nasal alar rim defects when additional support is needed. The typical donor site is from the anterior ear helix or the conchal bowl.

Cartilage graft is used when additional structure and support is needed. Typically, this involves larger defects involving the nose where the underlying cartilage is missing. The typical donor site is from the conchal bowl or ante-helix.

References

1.   Glogau RG, Haas AF. Skin Grafts. In: Baker SR, Swanson NA. Local Flaps in Facial Reconstruction. St. Louis: Mosby, Inc.; 1995. p. 247–71.
2.   Skouge JW. Skin grafting. New York: Churchill-Livingstone; 1991.

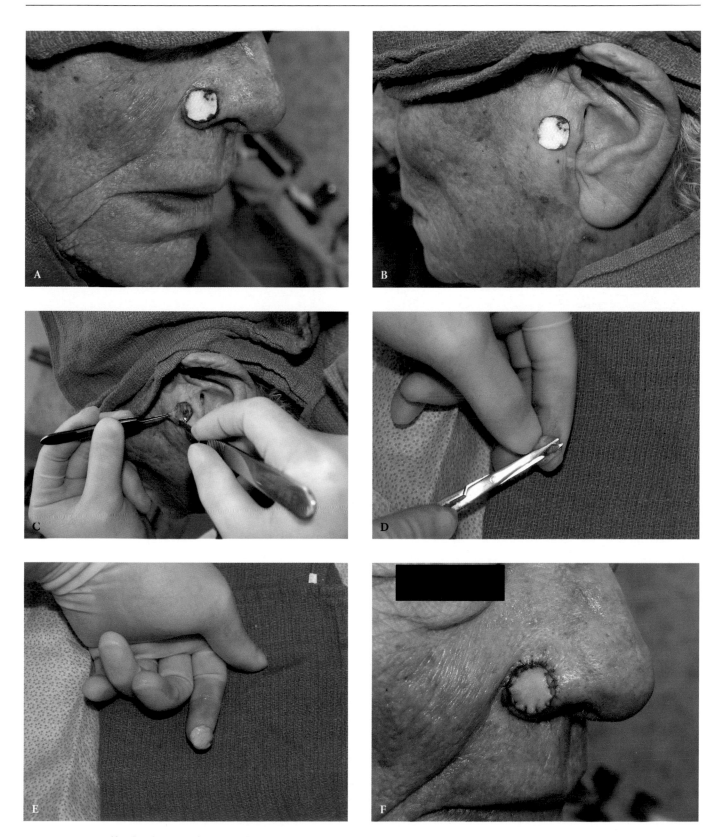

Figure 4.1 Full-Thickness Skin Graft (FTSG).

A. Template of a nasal ala defect is precisely made. The template should measure approximately 10% larger than the defect. **B.** The template is transferred to the donor site. **C.** Full thickness of the skin is excised in the shape of the template. **D.** The undersurface of the graft is trimmed of fat. **E.** The undersurface of the graft shows shiny dermis. **F.** The graft is carefully sutured into place. Bolster dressing is then applied on top of the graft.

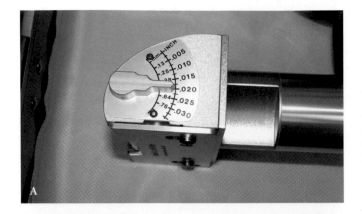

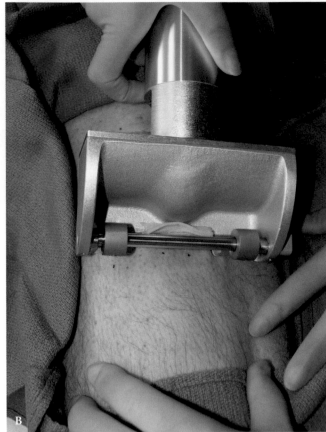

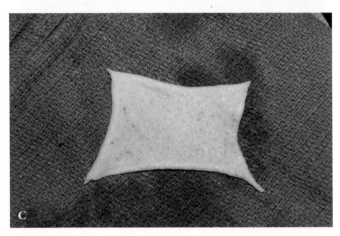

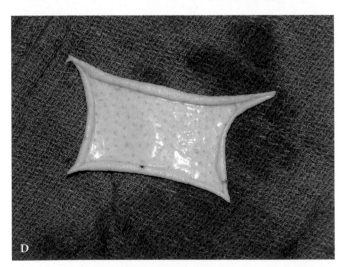

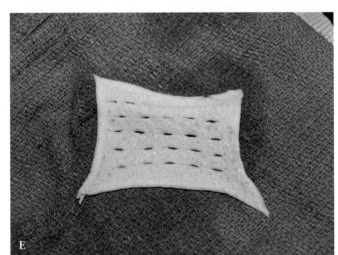

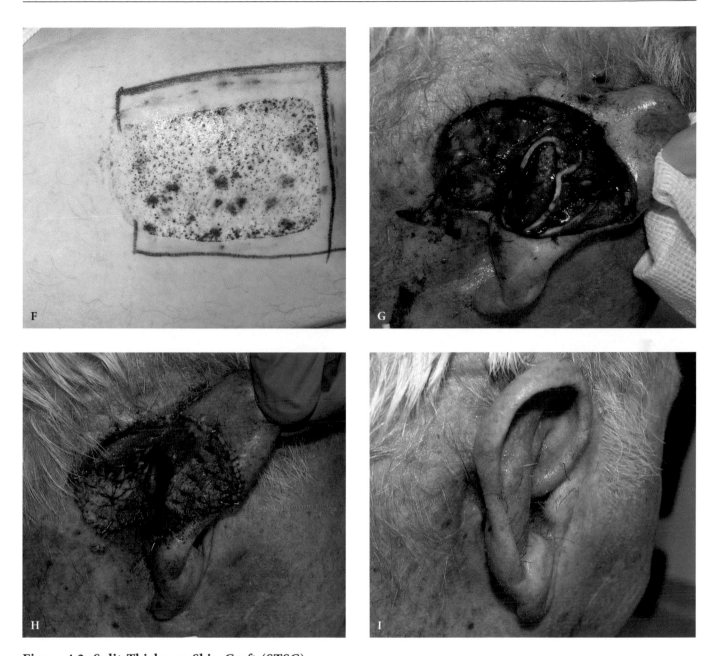

Figure 4.2 Split-Thickness Skin Graft (STSG).

A. Electric dermatome is set at the desired thickness of the graft. **B.** Small amount of mineral oil is applied to the skin. Traction is applied and the dermatome is firmly pressed against the skin at a 30–45° angle, then advanced forward resulting in the collection of the STSG. **C.** The epidermal surface has a dull appearance. **D.** The dermal surface has a shinier appearance. **E.** The graft is fenestrated to fit a larger defect. **F.** The donor site. **G.** Large defect on the posterior ear. **H.** STSG sutured in place. A bolster dressing is then applied on top of the graft. **I.** Four months post-op. The typical appearance is a depressed, hypopigmented, shiny graft.

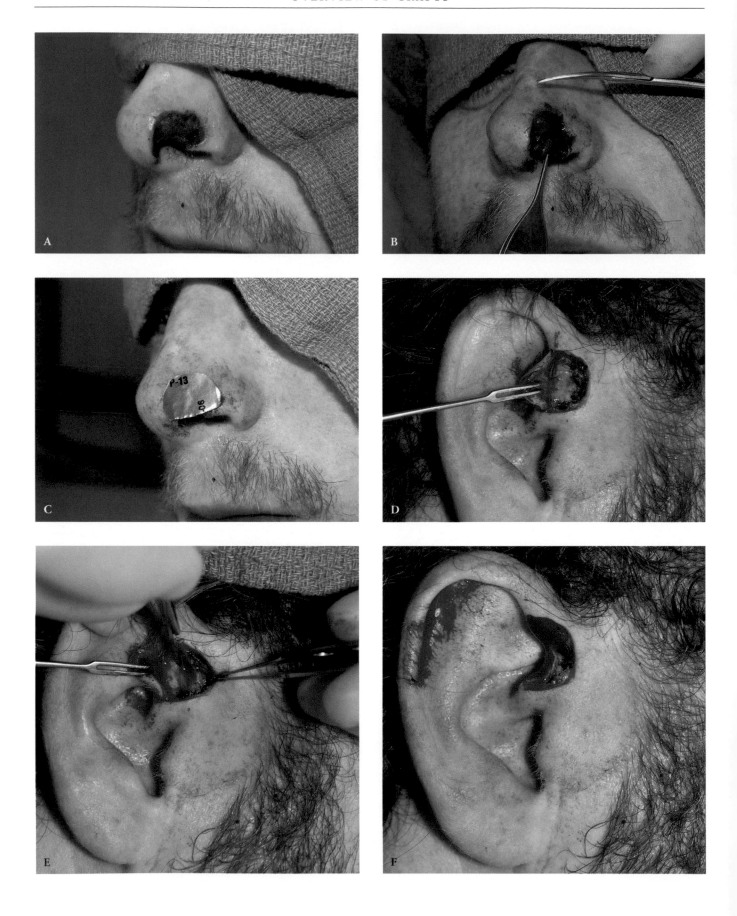

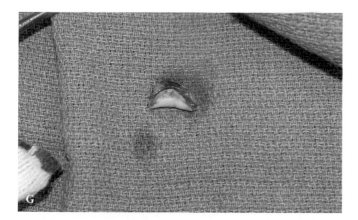

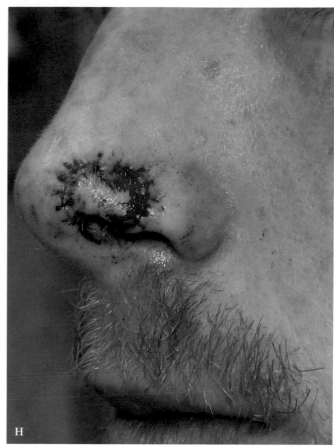

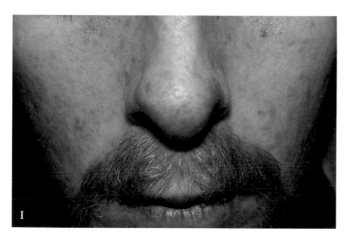

Figure 4.3 Composite Graft.

A. Defect involving the nasal ala and full thickness of the rim. **B.** The inner lining pulled down to create more "backboard" for the graft. **C.** Template placed on the defect. **D.** The skin portion excised from the anterior ear helix based on template. **E.** Incision is made through the cartilage. **F.** The remaining defect on the donor site is closed primarily in a linear fashion vertically. **G.** Composite graft with skin and attached cartilage. **H.** Graft sutured in place. **I.** Three months post-op. (Also see Chapter10, Figure 10.4)

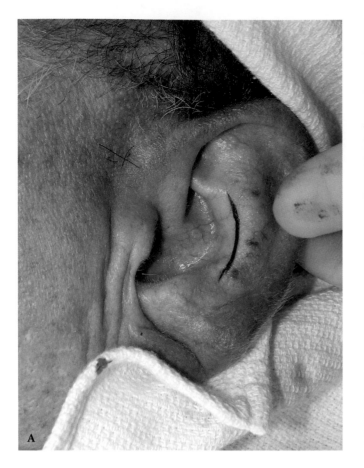

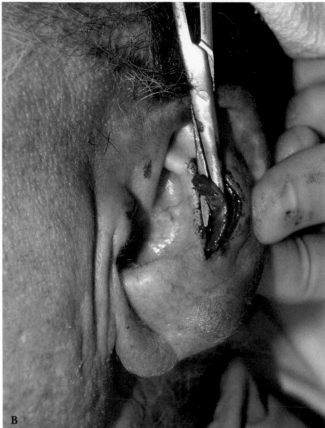

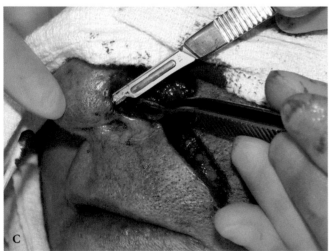

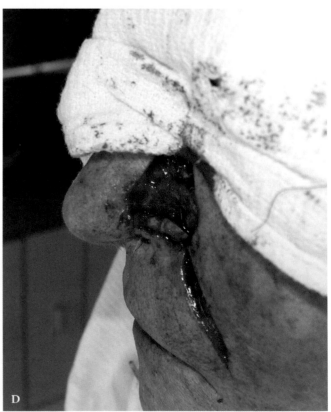

Figure 4.4 Cartilage Graft. Cartilage grafts are used to support the nasal ala and inserted inside of flaps.

A. Incision made on the skin of the ante-helix. **B.** Strip of cartilage is incised with a scalpel then carefully removed using scissors. **C.** Stab incisions are made on both ends where the graft will be inserted. **D.** The graft is inserted then secured by suture. (Also see Chapter 10, Figure 10.7)

CHAPTER 5

SCALP

The scalp represents one of the most homogenous and least complex anatomic regions of the head and neck. However, its unique characteristics and subtleties make reconstruction both challenging and rewarding. The broad, inelastic nature of the galea aponeurotica, which encompasses the scalp as a tendonlike sheath under constant tension, lends the scalp its less mobile characteristic. The anatomy is unlike any other, providing both benefits and drawbacks during reconstruction. Primary closures, flaps, and grafts may all be utilized to reconstruct the scalp, though their application can be very different when compared to other parts of the face. As such, and in comparison to facial skin, extensive undermining is often necessary during scalp reconstruction. The scalp is comprised of five layers: skin, subcutaneous connective tissue, galea, subaponeurotic loose areolar tissue, and pericranium. Scalp laxity can vary by age, location, and from person to person. Scalps in infants, for example, are quite loose and mobile. As one ages, this changes dramatically. The crown of the scalp usually is the least mobile, whereas the peripheral scalp is more distensible.

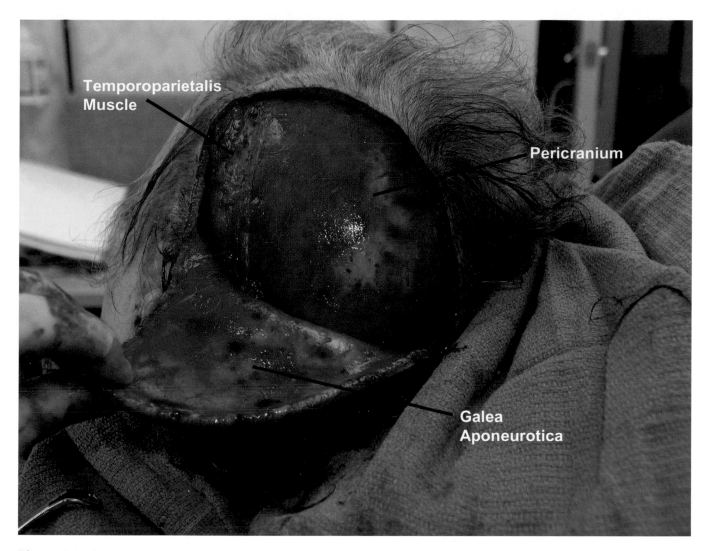

Figure 5.1 Anatomy.

Scalp flap is shown reflected at the level of the subgaleal plane. The flap contains the skin, subcutaneous fat, and galea. The base reveals loose areolar tissue, pericranium, and cranium. The temporoparietal muscle is located on the anteromedial aspect of the defect base. It is important to note that this muscle is deep to the galea as it is at the level of the muscles of mastication, thus differing from the frontalis and occipitalis muscles, which are enveloped by the galea at the level of the SMAS (superficial muscular aponeurotic system). Care must be taken in this area, and undermining in the subgaleal plane means staying above the temporoparietalis.

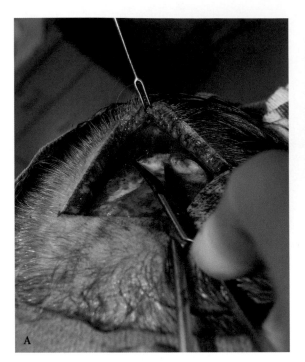 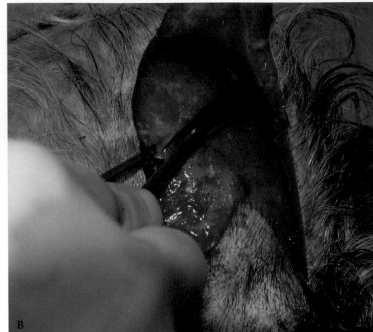

Figure 5.2 Undermining.

A. Undermining is performed in the subgaleal plane. The loose subaponeurotic connective tissue is easily separated by blunt dissection. **B.** Extensive undermining is needed on the scalp because of the inelasticity of the galea.

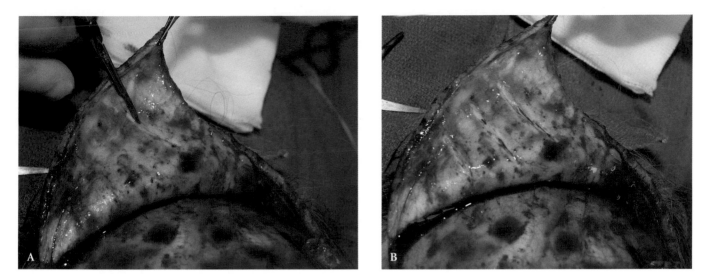

Figure 5.3 Galeotomy.

A, B. Using a scalpel blade, incisions are made on the undersurface of the galea in order to provide more mobility. The incision is oriented parallel to the leading edge of the flap and should be greater than 1 cm from the edge.

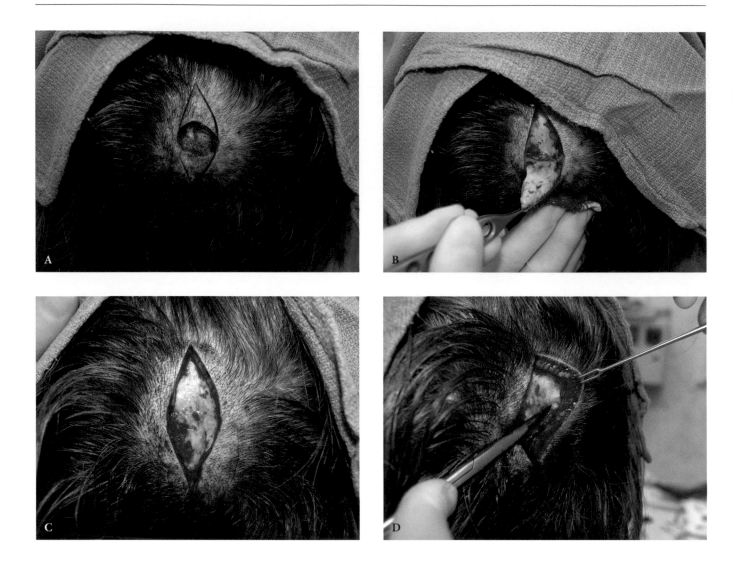

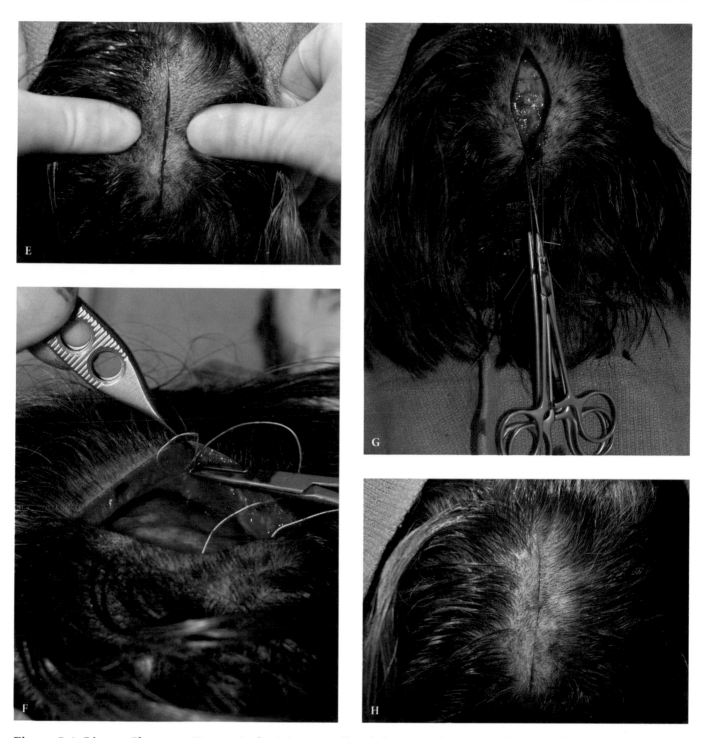

Figure 5.4 Linear Closure – Vertex Scalp. Many smaller defects can be repaired primarily.

A. Defect on the scalp vertex. Fusiform ellipse is oriented anteroposteriorly. **B.** The dog-ears and the base are removed at the level of the subgaleal plane. **C.** Defect to level of the pericranium. **D.** Undermining in the subgaleal plane. **E.** The undermining has sufficiently loosened the tissue so that it can be easily pushed together manually. **F.** Sutures are placed grabbing only the galea. **G.** In smaller defects, sutures are "tagged" with hemostats, which are not tied until the end, in order to facilitate the placement of the galeal sutures. **H.** Defect closed only with the galeal sutures. Note the tight approximation.

(Continued on next page.)

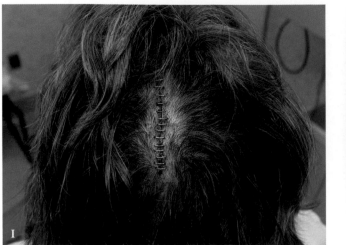
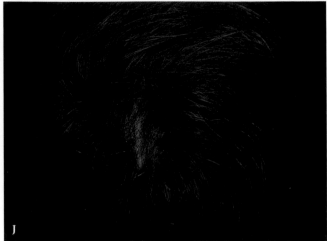

Figure 5.4 Linear Closure – Vertex Scalp *(continued)*.

I. Immediate post-op. Staples are practical for scalp closures, as they tangle less with hair. **J.** Nine months post-op.

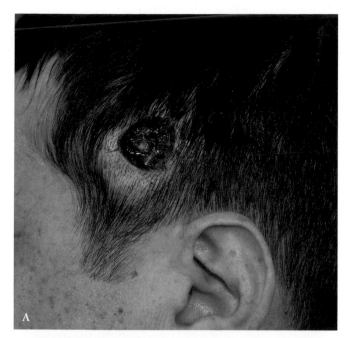

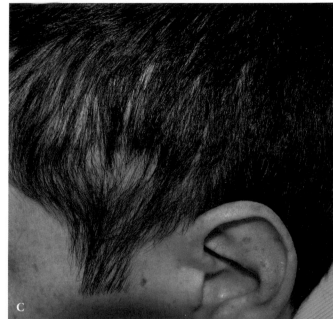

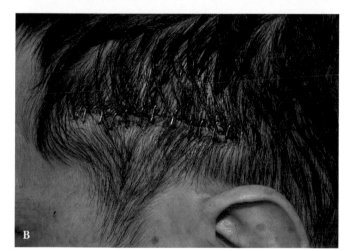

Figure 5.5 Linear Closure – Temporal Scalp.

A. Defect on the temporal scalp. **B.** The scar is oriented horizontally so that the hair that is superior to the scar will cover it. **C.** Six weeks post-op. Note that the hair is growing back to hide the scar.

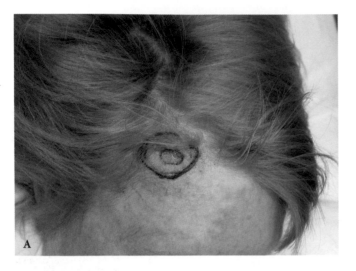
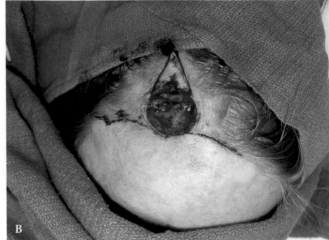
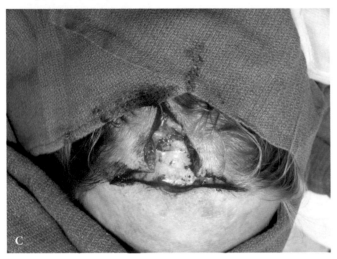
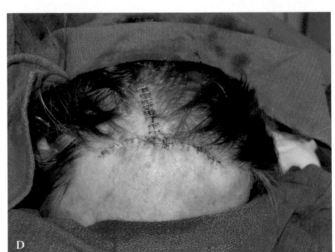
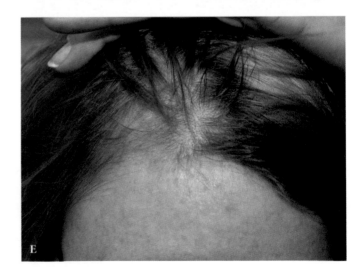

Figure 5.6 O-to-T Advancement Flap.

A. Outline of excision on the frontal scalp bordering the forehead. **B.** Defect with incision outline of the O-to-T advancement flap on the hairline. **C.** The defect extended through the galea and undermined in the subgaleal plane. **D.** Immediate post-op. **E.** Three months post-op. Note the regrowth of hair.

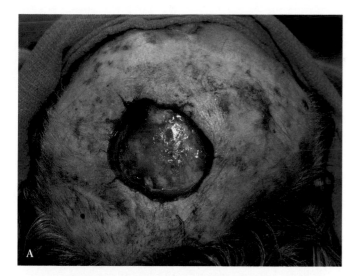

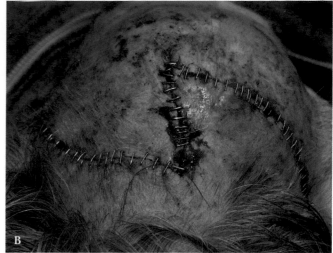

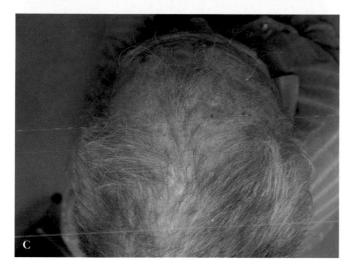

Figure 5.7 O-to-Z Rotation Flap. Rotation flaps are a mainstay of scalp reconstruction. The incisions need to be made much longer and a second rotation flap is sometimes added due to the stiffness of the scalp.

A. Defect on the vertex and frontal scalp. In the frontal scalp, the long incisions should be made parallel to the hairline so as not to extend on to the forehead. **B.** Immediate post-op. **C.** Five months post-op.

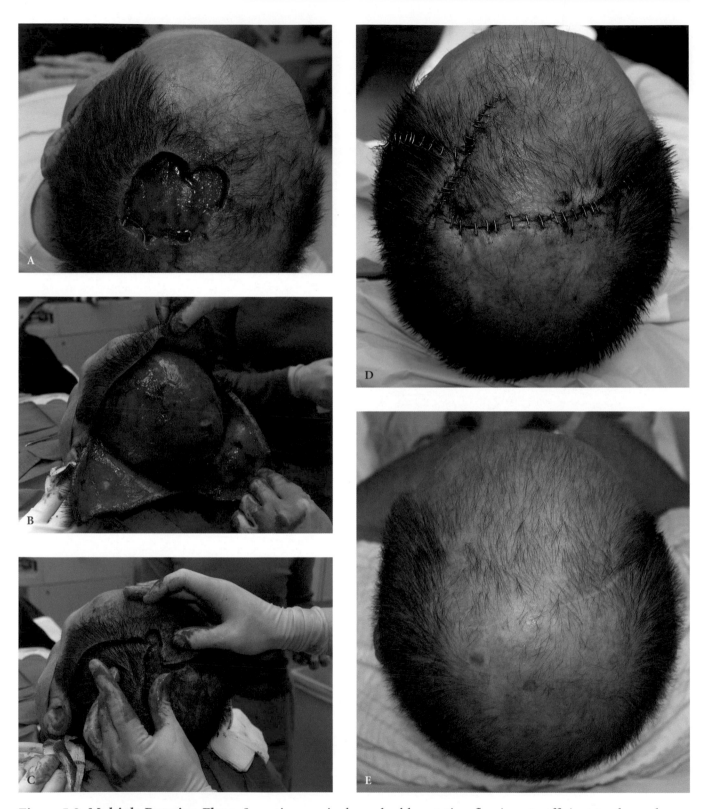

Figure 5.8 Multiple Rotation Flaps. Sometimes a single or double rotation flap is not sufficient to close a large or tight defect. Additional incisions are made to further mobilize the scalp.

A. Defect on the vertex and parietal scalp. **B.** Three long radial incisions equidistant on the perimeter of the defect. Flap reflected to show the extensive undermining necessary for the closure. **C.** Flap draped into place with minimal tension. **D.** Immediate post-op. When several radial incisions are made, it sometimes comes together in the shape of a pinwheel. It is not necessary, however, for the tips of the flaps to come together at one point. **F.** Two years post-op.

CHAPTER 6

FOREHEAD AND TEMPLE

The forehead and temple possess many characteristics similar to the scalp, though the reconstruction can often be quite different. The frontalis muscle is enveloped by the galea aponeurotica, though the mobility is greater than that of the scalp. The frontalis ends laterally at the temple and is replaced by fascia. The temporal branch of the facial nerve courses under the thin fascia, and therefore is particularly vulnerable with no overlying muscle to protect the nerve.

Most small forehead defects should be repaired in the horizontal direction parallel to the forehead creases. This becomes more difficult to accomplish as defects become larger, as there is more tension and eyebrow elevation. Smaller defects can be closed undermining in the subcutaneous fat, where there is less risk of nerve injury and greater tissue mobility. With larger defects, wide undermining in this plane becomes more difficult because the skin is quite adherent to the underlying frontalis muscle. The frontalis muscle fibers run in vertical direction; therefore, one must be careful not to tear through the muscle when reapproximating in a horizontal direction.

Larger defects are closed in the vertical direction with the tension vector aligned horizontally and undermined in the avascular subfrontalis plane. Because of the laxity, vertical scars heal very well with minimal spread.

Temple defects are often closed with skin movement from the looser cheek skin. By hiding much of the scar line in the hair or hairline, large defects can be closed with inconspicuous scars. Temple defects can sometimes be allowed to heal by second intent. Because of the concavity of this region, a depressed scar that results from granulation blends in well.

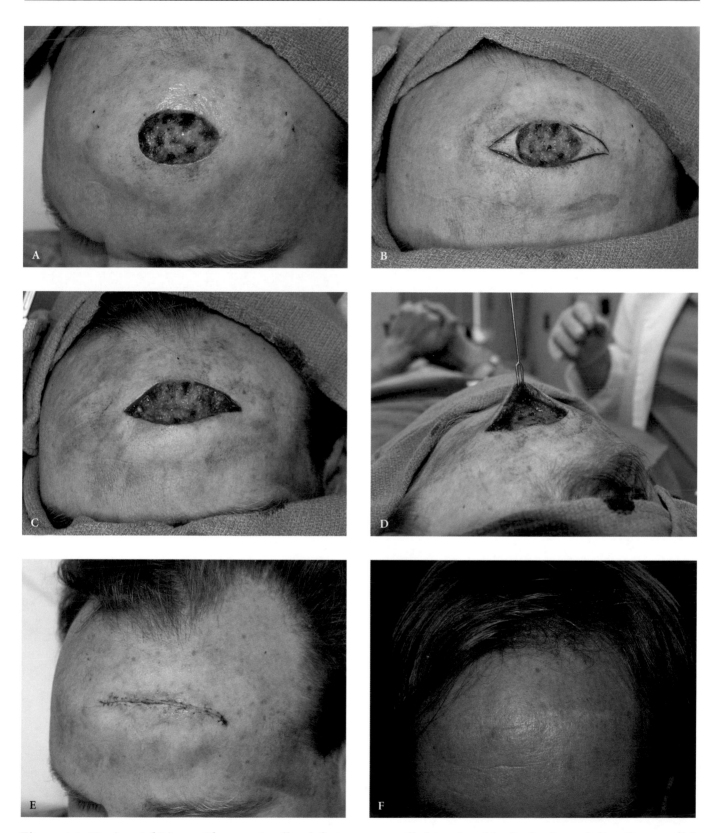

Figure 6.1 Horizontal Linear Closure. Smaller defects are generally best closed in the horizontal direction parallel to the forehead creases.

(Continued on next page.)

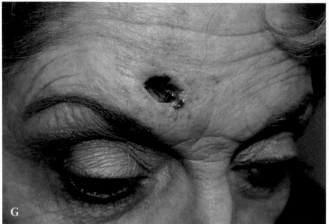

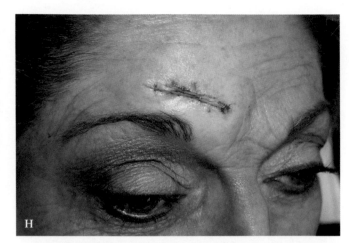

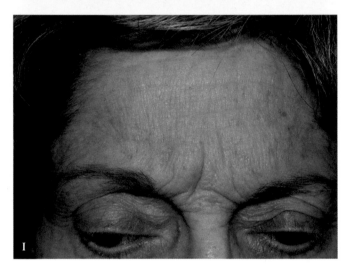

Figure 6.1 Horizontal Linear Closure *(continued).*

A. Defect on the upper forehead. This is probably the maximal size for a horizontal closure. **B, C.** Dog-ears removed to shape the scar in a slightly curvilinear fashion. **D.** Undermining in the subcutaneous fat. Compared to undermining in the subfrontalis muscle plane, there is less brow elevation. **E.** Immediate post-op. Running horizontal sutures used for the cuticular layer. Wound edges must be well everted in this region or the scar will indent into the forehead crease. **F.** One year post-op. **G, H.** Near the eyebrow, the forehead crease is not horizontal. **I.** Four months post-op.

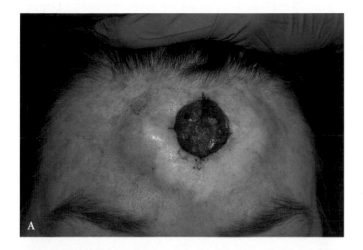

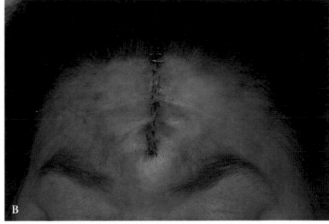

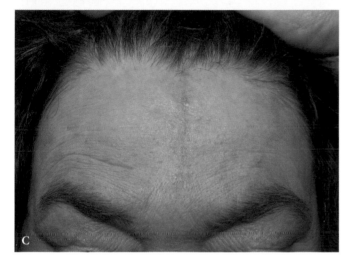

Figure 6.2 Vertical Linear Closure. Medium- to large-size defects close more easily in the vertical direction.

A. Defect on the forehead. **B.** Immediate post-op, undermined in the subcutaneous fat. **C.** Two months post-op.

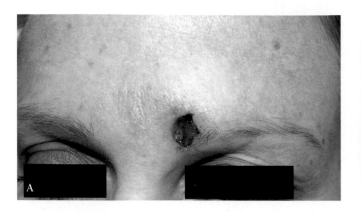

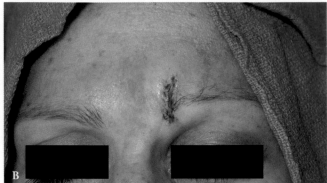

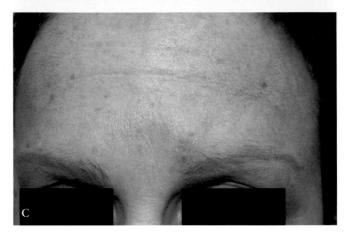

Figure 6.3 Vertical Linear Closure.

A. Defect involving the medial eyebrow. **B.** The defect is repaired with careful reapproximating the eyebrow. **C.** One-month post-op.

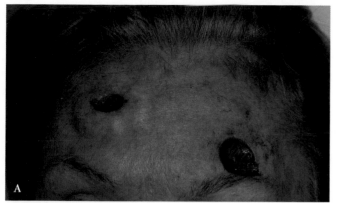

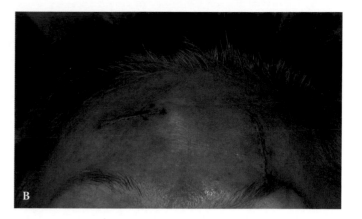

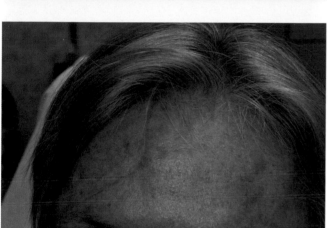

Figure 6.4 O-to-L Advancement Flap and Linear Closure.

A. Two defects – superior forehead and forehead above eyebrow. **B.** Immediate post-op. O-to-L advancement flap is used to keep the incision along the superior eyebrow junction. The superior defect is repaired with linear closure along the crease. **C.** Six months post-op.

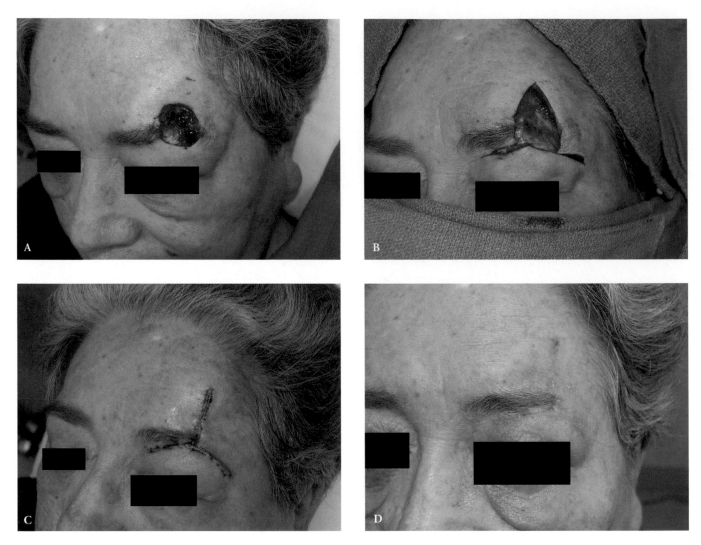

Figure 6.5 O-to-T Advancement Flap of the Eyebrow. O-to-L is converted to O-to-T when additional movement is needed.

A. Defect on the lateral eyebrow and forehead. **B.** O-to-T advancement flap, designed with the horizontal component along the inferior eyebrow border. **C.** Immediate post-op. The remaining eyebrow margins are carefully approximated. **D.** Two months post-op. The O-T takes advantage of the ease of closing in the vertical direction and blending into cosmetic junctions.

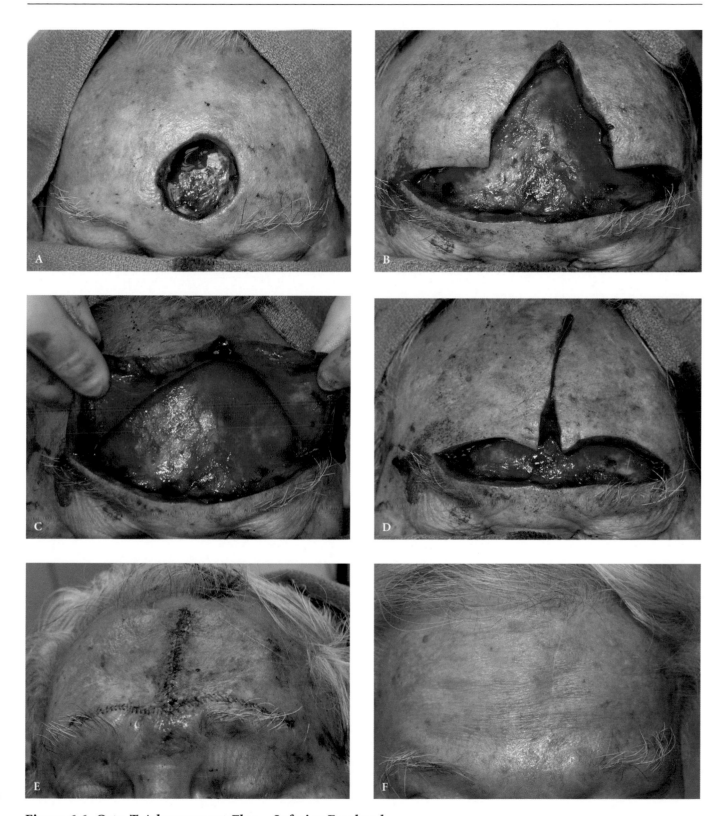

Figure 6.6 O-to-T Advancement Flap – Inferior Forehead.

A. Defect through the frontalis muscle. **B.** Incisions made horizontally in line with the eyebrows and dog-ear removed superiorly. **C.** Undermining in the subfrontalis (subgaleal) plane. **D.** Vertical incision closed first with careful reapproximation of the frontalis muscle. **E.** Immediate post-op. The horizontal incision is curved slightly to better blend with the eyebrow margin. **F.** Three-month follow-up.

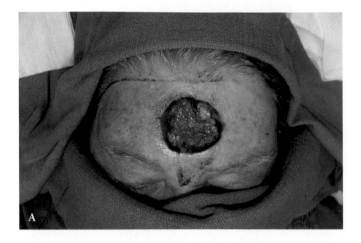

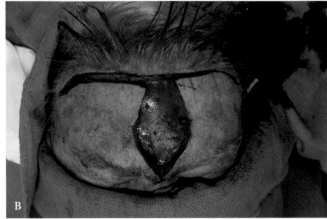

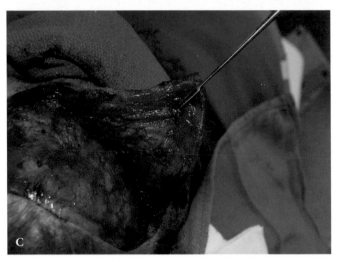

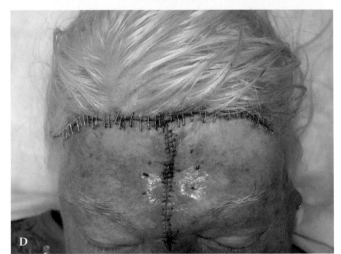

Figure 6.7 O-to-T Advancement Flap – Superior Forehead.

A. Defect through the frontalis muscle. **B.** Defect extended up to the hairline. Incisions made horizontally along the hairline. **C.** Undermining in the subfrontalis (subgaleal) plane with galeotomies. **D.** Immediate post-op. **E.** Five weeks post-op. Note that the frontalis muscle is functional.

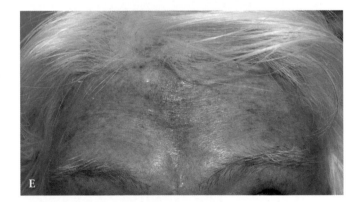

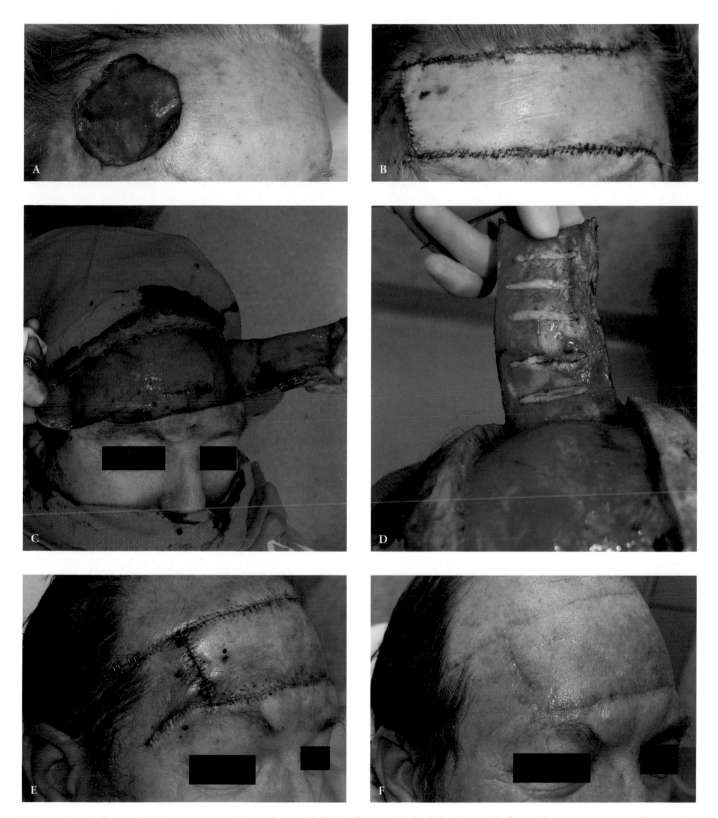

Figure 6.8 Bilateral Advancement Flap, also called H-plasty, is ideal for large defects that encompass the entire vertical height of the forehead.

A. Large defect on the lateral forehead, extending from eyebrow to frontal hairline. **B.** Immediate post-op. The H is asymmetric because the defect is not central. **C.** Another defect with the flap reflected back at the level of the subfrontalis plane. **D.** Galeotomies to increase flap mobility. **E.** Immediate post-op. **F.** One month post-op.

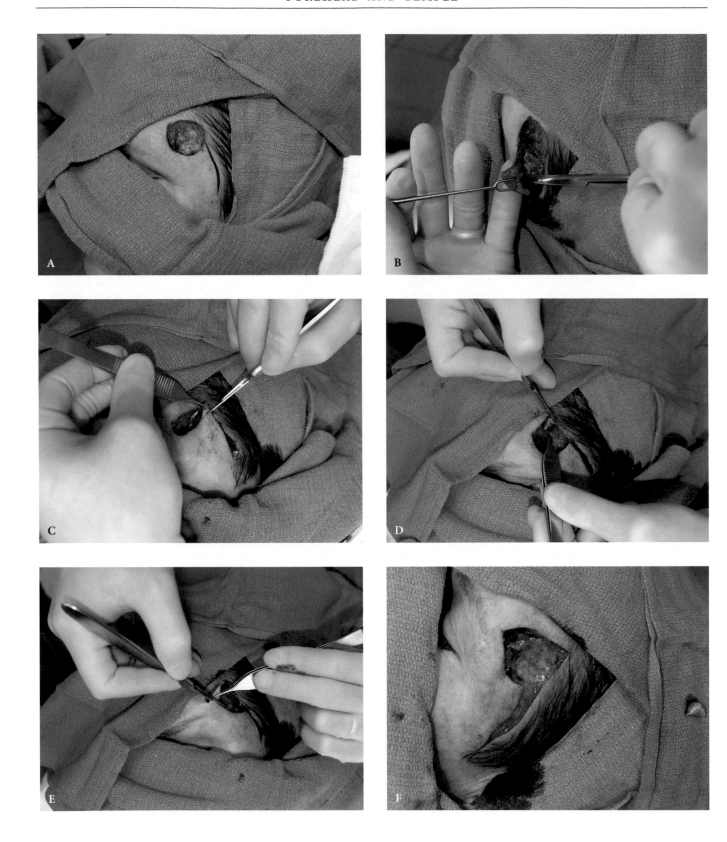

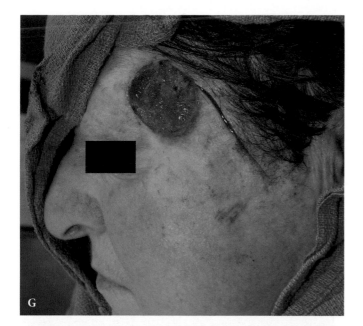

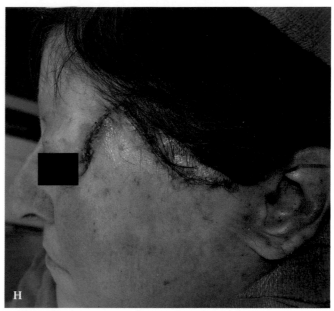

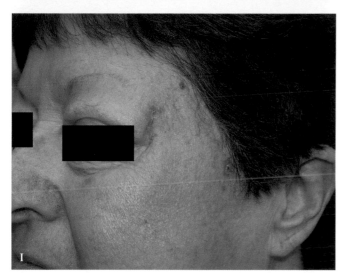

Figure 6.9 Temple-Advancement Flap. Defects on the temple can be repaired with an advancement flap with much of the scar hidden in the hairline.

A. Defect on the temple with incision along the hairline. **B.** Flap undermined in the subcutaneous fat plane. The temporal branch of the facial nerve traverses this anatomic region, protected only by the superficial fascia. **C–F.** The flap tip and the round defect are squared off by the removal of dog-ears. **G.** Similar defect with incision placed along hairline. **H.** Immediate post-op. The inferior dog-ear is taken posteriorly, to be hidden in the sideburn. **I.** Six-week post-op. Note that the distortion and elevation of the eyelid/brow have resolved.

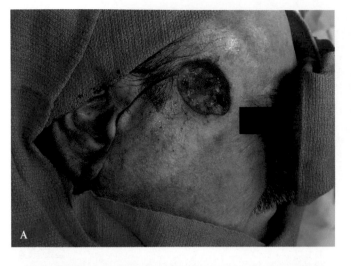

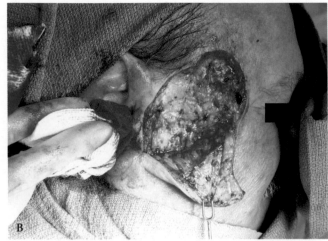

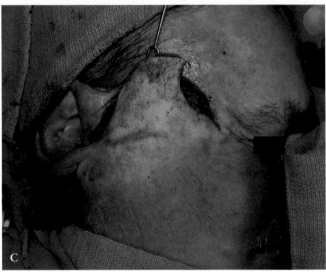

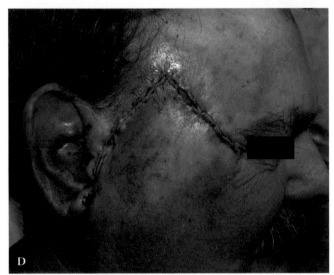

Figure 6.10 Temple-Advancement Flap 2.

A. Larger defect extending into the scalp. Incision is made within the scalp and extended posterior to the sideburn. **B.** Flap is undermined and lifted in the subcutaneous plane. **C.** Flap is draped into position. **D.** Immediate post-op. The incision was extended inferiorly along the preauricular sulcus. Most of the scar is hidden and the distortion has resolved. **E.** One month post-op.

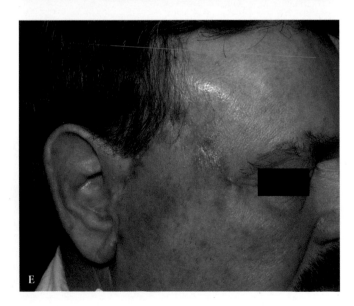

CHAPTER 7

CHEEK

The cheek is anatomically defined by the nasofacial sulcus and the melolabial folds medially, the preauricular sulcus laterally, the orbital rim and zygomatic arch superiorly, and the jawline inferiorly. At first, cheeks may appear to be one of the easiest areas to perform facial surgery. In fact, it may be one of the least forgiving. There are no cosmetic junctions and creases within the cheek to hide the incisions.

The use of the relaxed skin tension lines is probably more important in the cheeks than any other area on the face for this reason, especially in younger patients where wrinkles are absent. Precise markings of the relaxed skin tension lines will yield better results.

The cheek may appear to be topographically flat, but there are contours that should be preserved for optimal symmetry. Careful attention to the three-dimensional quality of the malar cheek is important, as oftentimes surgery can flatten it.

Some general rules for cheek reconstruction:

If the defect can be closed primarily in a linear or curvilinear fashion along the relaxed skin tension lines, do so.

Place the incisions either along the cosmetic borders of the cheeks, or on the lateral portion of the cheek (where it is less visible from the front).

The neck skin is a great reservoir for skin mobility.

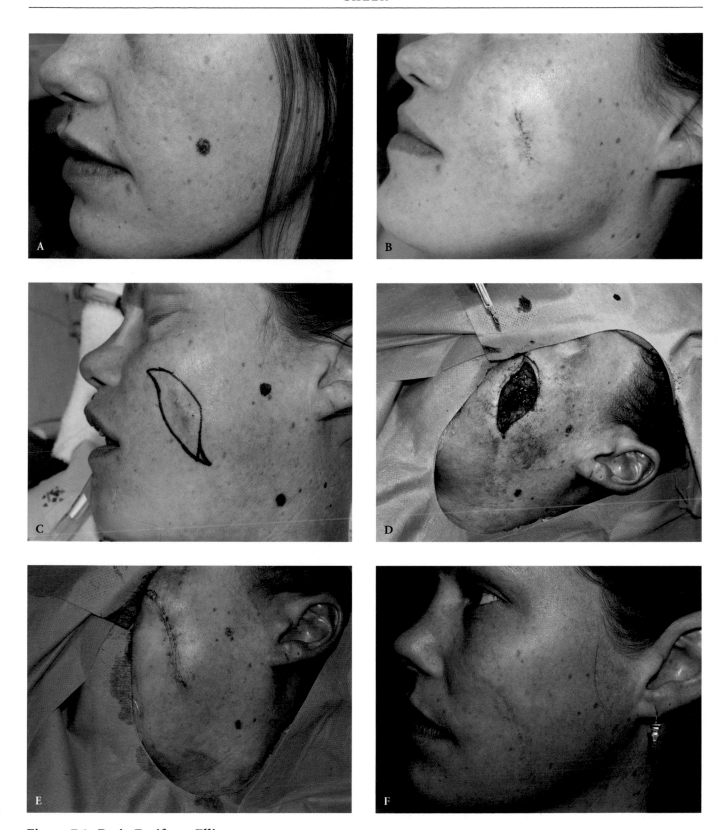

Figure 7.1 Basic Fusiform Ellipse.

A. Lesion on the cheek suspicious of malignant melanoma. **B.** Basic excisional biopsy along the relaxed skin tension line. **C.** Wide local excision of melanoma outlined along relaxed skin tension line in fusiform ellipse with a Lazy-S modificiation. **D.** Defect post wide local excision. The blue represents the dye used for sentinel lymph node biopsy. **E.** Immediate post-op. **F.** Nine months post-op.

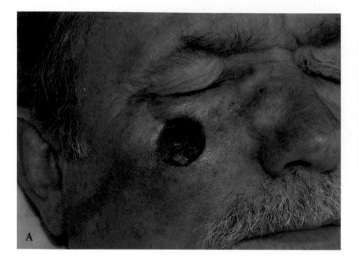

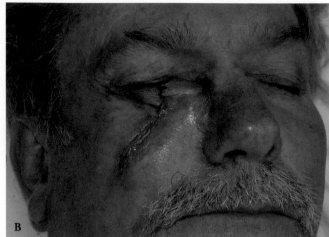

Figure 7.2 Linear Closure.

A. Defect on the right-upper cheek. **B.** Linear closure in a lazy-S curvilinear fashion along the relaxed skin tension line. The lazy-S shape is particularly suited for convexities to minimize blunting. **C.** Six-month post-op.

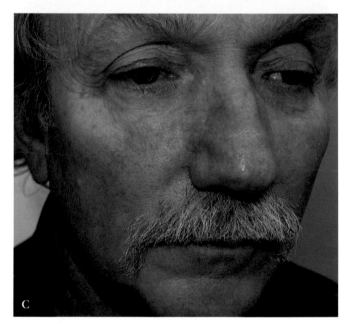

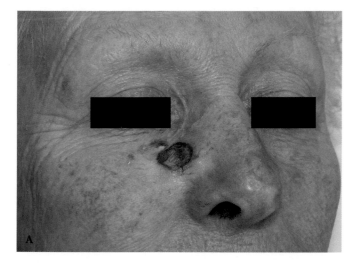

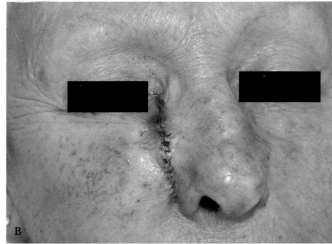

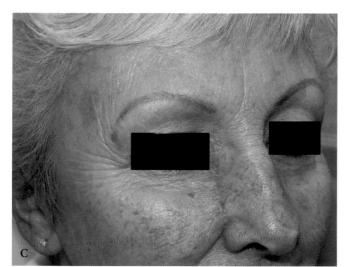

Figure 7.3 Linear Closure.

A. Defect on the nasofacial sulcus. **B.** Although this may not fit precisely within the relaxed skin tension lines, the incision line is placed in the cosmetic junction. **C.** Six weeks post-op.

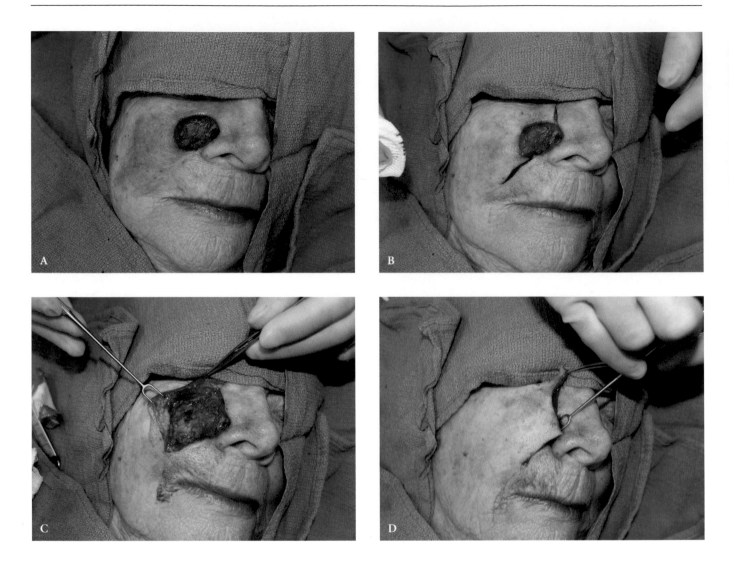

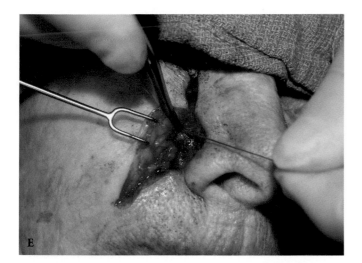

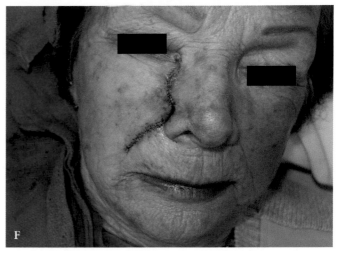

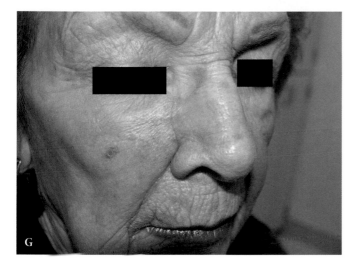

Figure 7.4 Advancement Flap – Medial Cheek.

A. A defect on the medial cheek abutting the nasofacial sulcus and nasal alar crease is ideal for this flap.
B. Incisions are made superiorly and inferiorly on the cosmetic junctions. **C.** Flap is undermined widely in the subcutaneous plane, leaving most of the malar fat pad intact at the base of the defect. It is important not to push the fat medially, as this will flatten the cheek. **D.** Adequately undermined flap is draped into position. **E.** As this defect extended onto the nose inferiorly, the flap is tacked to the periosteum to prevent tenting. **F.** Immediate post-op. The portion at the alar crease is allowed to heal by second intent in order to recreate the convexity. **G.** Six weeks post-op.

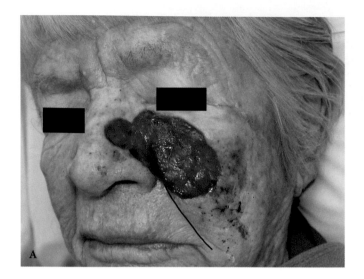

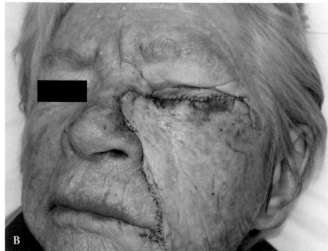

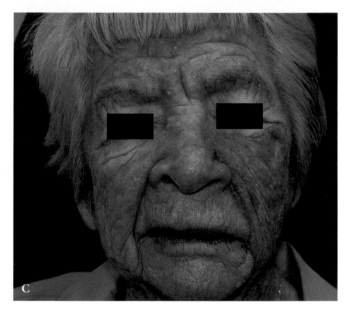

Figure 7.5 Advancement Flap – Inferiorly Based.

A. Broad defect on the medial cheek. Because of the width of the defect, it would be difficult to advance skin laterally. In older patients, there is usually ample laxity inferiorly. The incision is made along the melolabial crease inferiorly. **B.** Immediate post-op. The flap is widely undermined and advanced far enough superiorly so that there is no tension on the lower eyelid. The placement of periosteal sutures on the lateral orbital rim and nasal bone also helps to support the flap. **C.** Six weeks post-op. Note the lack of tension on the lower eyelid and the restoration of the cheek symmetry.

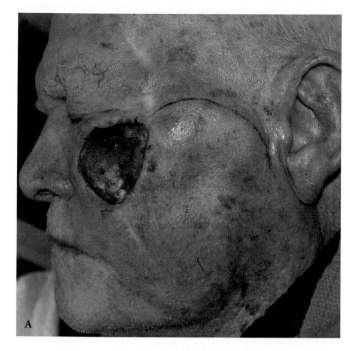

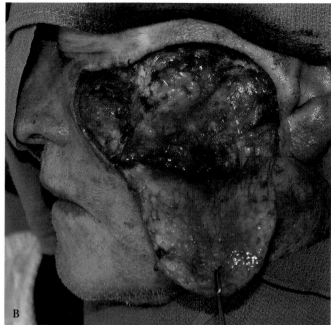

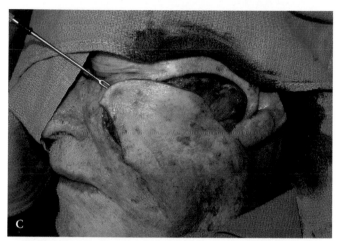

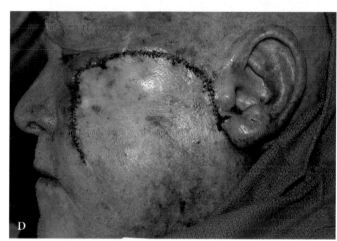

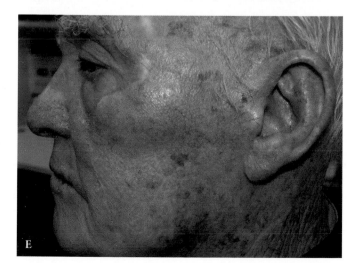

Figure 7.6 Rotation Flap.

A. Defect on the central cheek. The rotation flap is drawn so that the incision arcs superiorly above the lateral canthus in order to prevent ectropion. **B.** The flap is incised, undermined in the subcutaneous fat plane, and reflected. **C.** Flap draped into position. **D.** Immediate post-op. Burow's triangle is taken out behind the ear. **E.** Six weeks post-op.

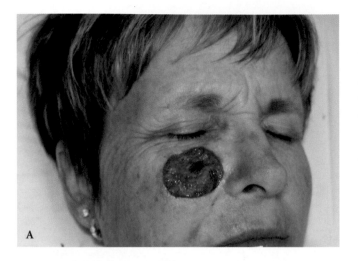

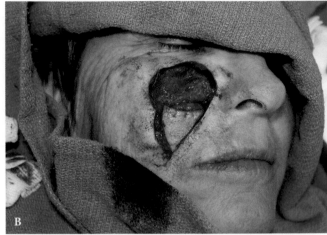

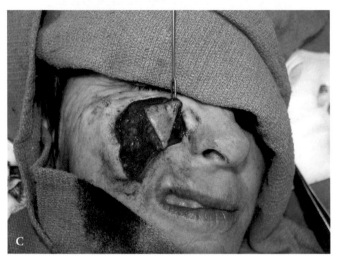

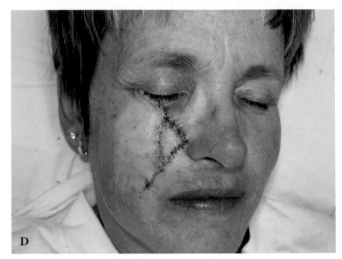

Figure 7.7 Island Pedicle Flap.

A. Defect on the medial cheek extending onto the nasal sidewall. A primary closure would likely blunt the cheek and melolabial fold. **B.** Island pedicle flap is designed inferiorly with the incision along the melolabial fold. **C.** The flap is raised with the pedicle attached at the base and draped into position. **D.** Immediate post-op. **E.** Four-month post-op. Island pedicle flaps have a tendency to trap-door, which in this case helps to recreate the cheek convexity.

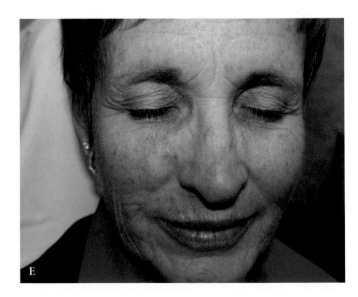

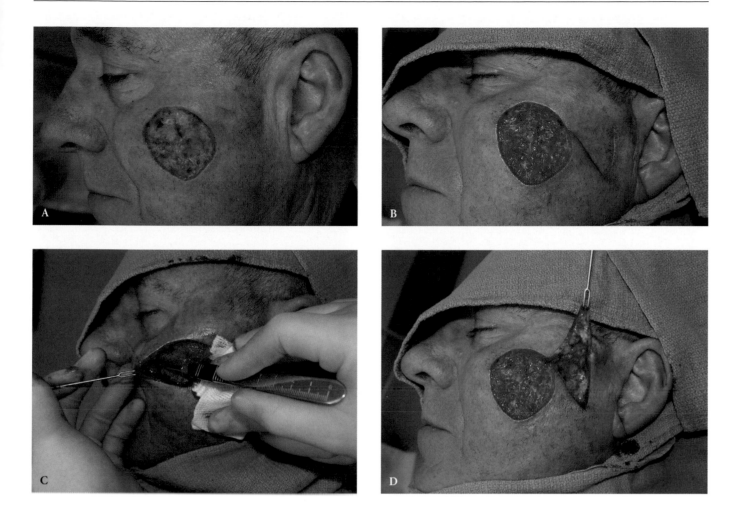

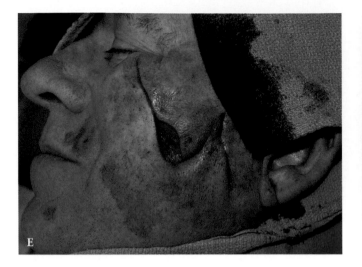

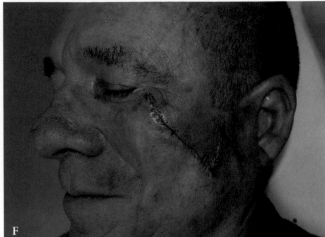

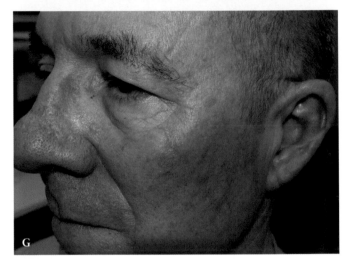

Figure 7.8 Rhombic Transposition Flap.

A. Defect on lateral cheek. **B.** Modified rhombic transposition flap is designed inferiorly and laterally to the defect from an area of greatest tissue laxity. **C.** Wide undermining around the defect in order to facilitate secondary motion from the medial direction and minimize trap-door effect. **D.** Flap is elevated. **E.** The secondary defect is sutured first then the flap is transposed into the primary defect. **F.** Immediate post-op. **G.** Six weeks post-op.

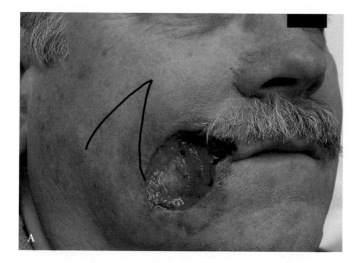

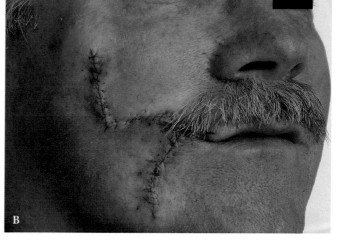

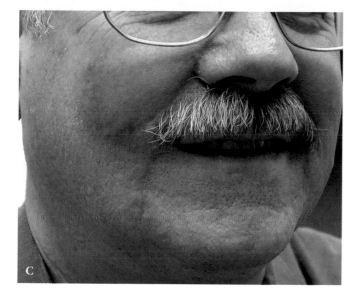

Figure 7.9 Rhombic Transposition Flap.

A. Defect on the lower medial cheek. **B.** Rhombic flap designed superiorly. Note that the incision lines parallel the relaxed skin tension lines. **C.** One-month post-op.

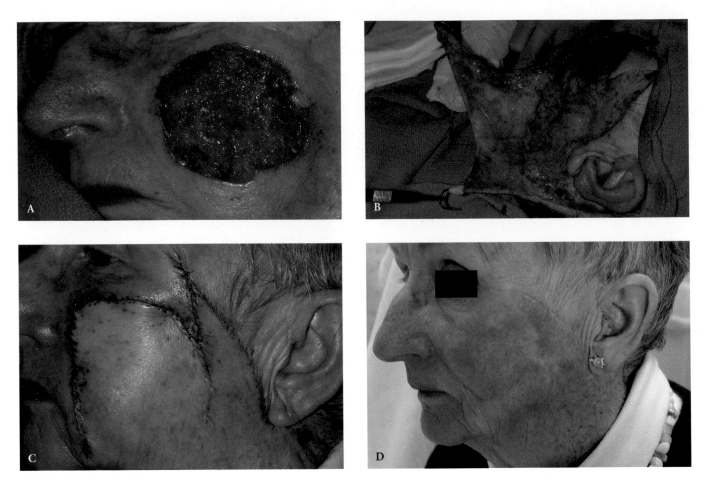

Figure 7.10 Bilobe Flap.

A. Large defect on the central cheek, which would be difficult to close with a rhombic flap. Bilobe flap is designed with the primary lobe from the lateral cheek and the secondary lobe from behind the ear. **B.** Flap incised, undermined, and reflected. **C.** Immediate post-op. **D.** One year post-op.

CHAPTER 8

EYELID

The eyelids extend from the eyelid margins to involve all the skin within the orbital rim. In reconstructing the eyelids, both the functional and cosmetic aspects must carefully be taken into consideration. Symmetry is paramount in achieving optimal cosmetic results. Of equal or greater importance is the functional restoration of the eyelid. The sphincter action of the orbicularis oculi muscle needs to be preserved for normal opening and closing of the eyelids. Furthermore, vector tensions on the lower eyelid must be carefully considered in order to prevent ectropia.

The anatomy and reconstruction of the eyelid can be quite complex.

There are, however, few important points that can simplify this process.

- Reapproximate each anatomic structure, for example, tarsus, orbicularis, lid margin.
- Design flaps that give an upward tension vector on the lower lid.
- Oversize grafts and flaps for the lower lid.
- Generally, align linear closures in a more vertical orientation, perpendicular to the lower-eyelid margin.

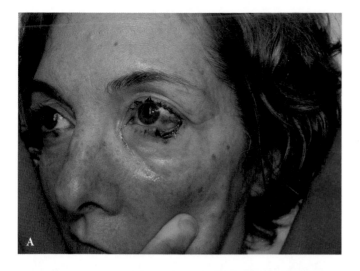

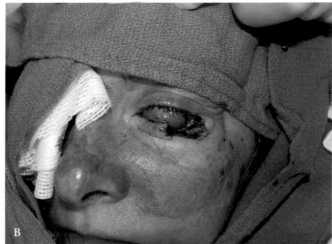

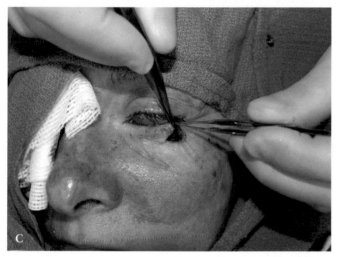

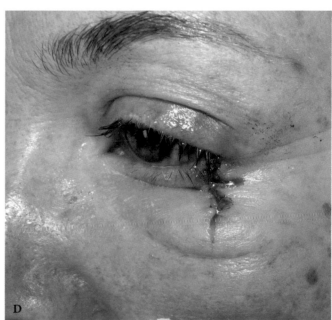

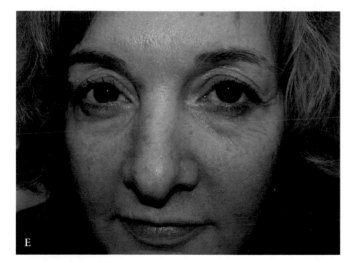

Figure 8.1 Wedge Repair of Lower Eyelid.

A. Full thickness defect involving one-third of the lower eyelid. This is close to the maximum defect size that can be repaired with a simple wedge without a canthal release. **B.** Full thickness dog-ear is removed. Each of these exposed layers must be carefully re-approximated. Tarsus, eyelid margin, orbicularis oculi, and skin. **C.** The eyelid margins are temporarily reapproximated with forceps to assess mobility. **D.** Immediate post-op. **E.** Two months post-op. Note the symmetry.

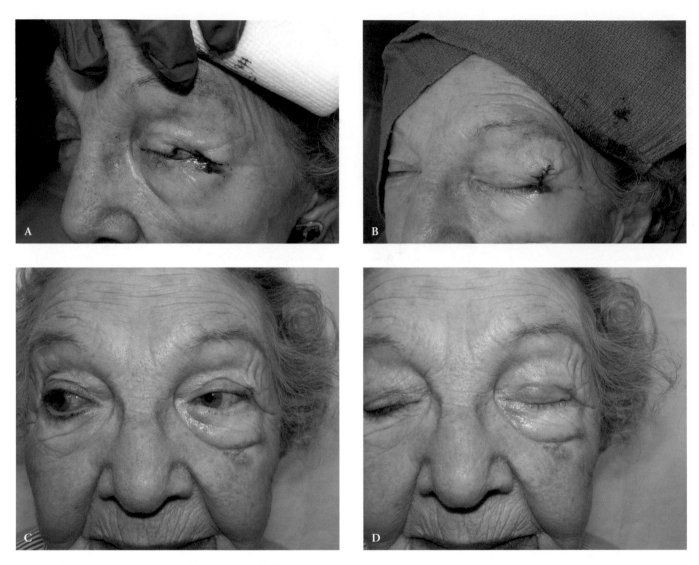

Figure 8.2 Wedge Repair of Upper Eyelid.

A. Full thickness defect involving one-third of the upper eyelid. **B.** Immediate post-op. Full thickness dog-ear is removed. Each of these exposed layers are carefully reapproximated. Tarsus, eyelid margin, orbicularis oculi, and skin. **C, D.** One month post-op.

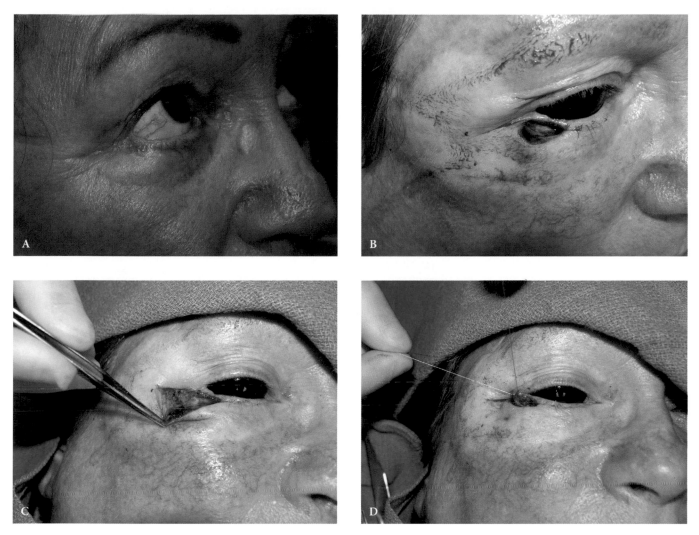

Figure 8.3 Lateral Canthal Tendon Plication. (Canthopexy) This technique is helpful in both the repair of minor ectropion and tightening of a lax lower eyelid in conjunction with other repairs.

A. Preoperative photo of recurrent basal cell carcinoma from previous wedge excision. Note the thinning and indentation of the eyelid margin. **B.** Defect through the orbicularis oculi muscle. **C.** Incision extended along the subciliary line, then slightly superior, lateral to the lateral canthus without its disruption. **D.** The lateral canthal tendon is grasped with suture.

(Continued on next page.)

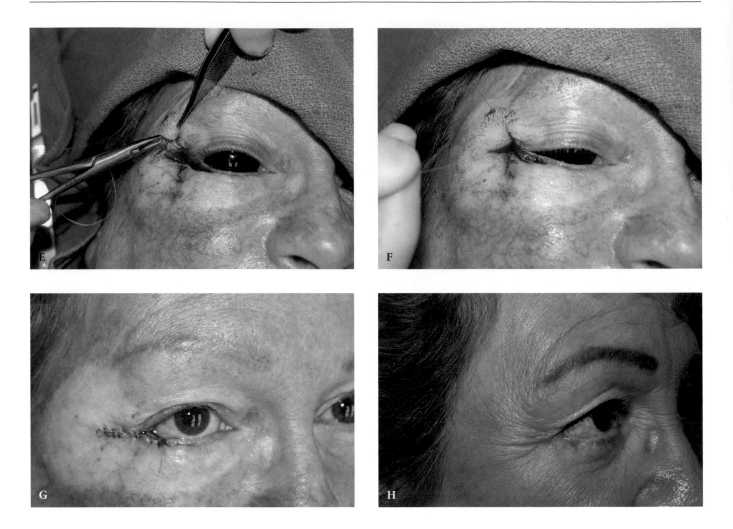

Figure 8.3 Lateral Canthal Tendon Plication. *(continued).*

E. The needle is passed through the periosteum of the orbital rim beneath the lateral canthus. **F.** The suture is secured to the periosteum and then tied. Note the superior and posterior movement of the lower lid. **G.** Immediate post-op. The lower-lid skin is re-approximated. **H.** Two-month follow-up. Note the similar position of the lower-eyelid margin to the preoperative photo (Figure 8.3A).

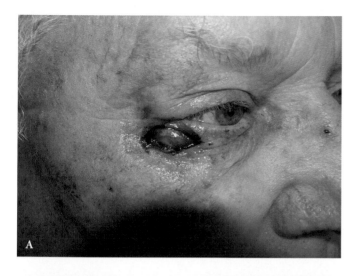

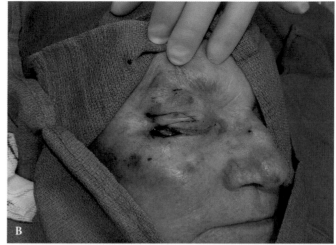

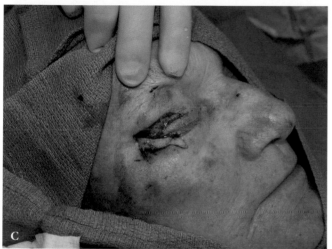

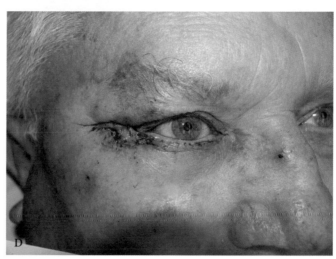

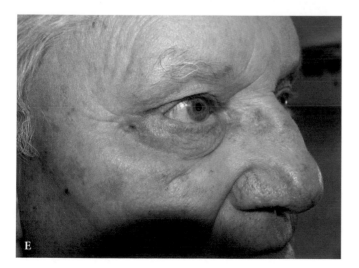

Figure 8.4 Cross lid transposition flap.

A. Defect of the lower lateral eyelid. **B.** Banner type transposition flap incised on the upper eyelid. **C.** Flap lifted and transposed to the lower-lid defect. **D.** Flap sutured into place. Lateral canthal tendon was also plicated. **E.** Two months post-op.

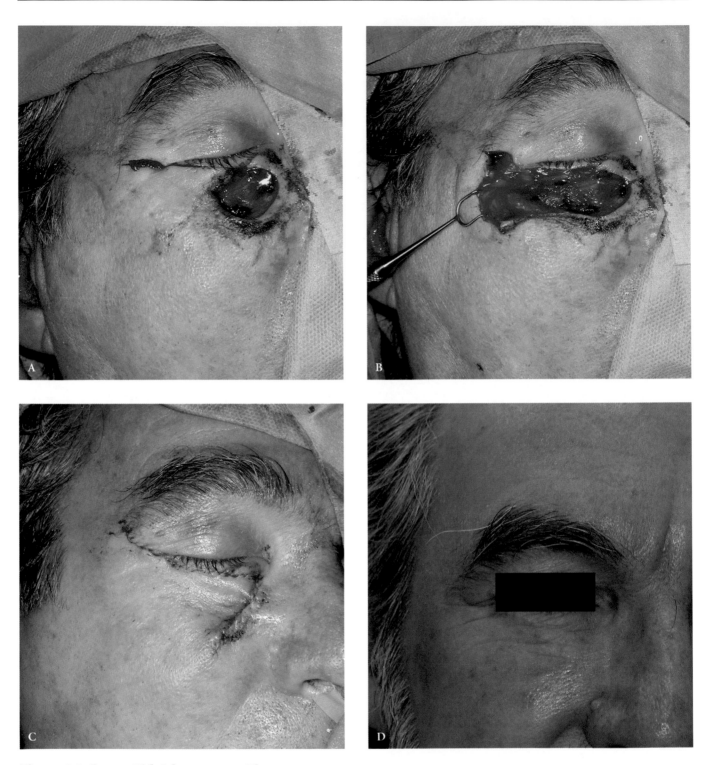

Figure 8.5 Lower-Lid Advancement Flap.

A. Defect of the lower lateral eyelid. Incision made from the defect to the subciliary line and then superiorly above the level of the lateral canthus. The placement above the level of the canthus is the key step as it provides an upward tension vector to prevent an ectropion. **B.** Flap undermined and lifted. **C.** Immediate post-op. **D.** Two months post-op.

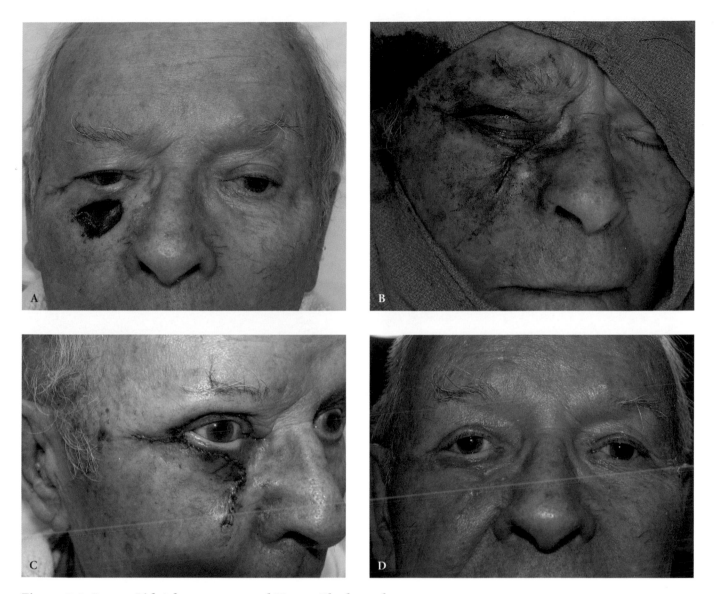

Figure 8.6 Lower-Lid Advancement and Upper Blepharoplasty.

A. Defect of the lower-eyelid skin. Note the lower-eyelid laxity and asymmetric upper-eyelid hooding. **B.** Flap advanced into place and lower-lid laxity removed with lateral canthal tendon plication. Excess upper eyelid skin removed. **C.** Immediate post-op. **D.** One month post-op.

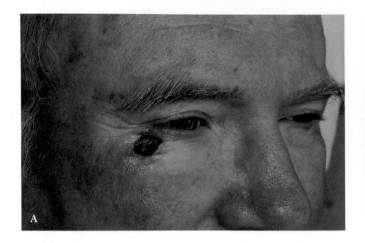

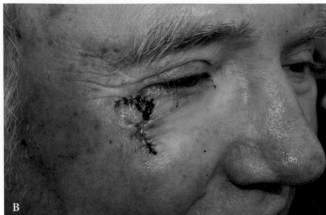

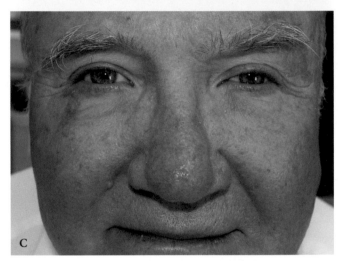

Figure 8.7 Rhombic Transposition Flap of the Lower Lid.

A. Lower-lid defect. **B.** Immediate post-op. Oversized rhombic flap is transposed into place in order to prevent a downward pull. **C.** One month post-op.

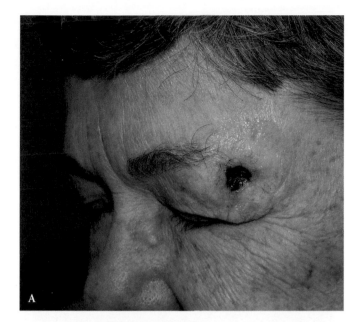

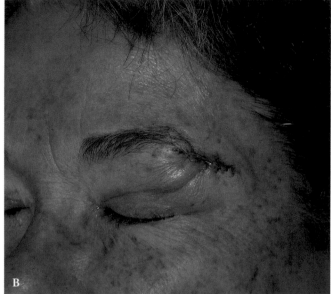

Figure 8.8 Upper Lid Linear Repair. Small defects on the upper lid can be closed in a horizontal direction.

A. Defect on the upper lateral eyelid. **B.** Immediate post-op. **C.** Six months post-op.

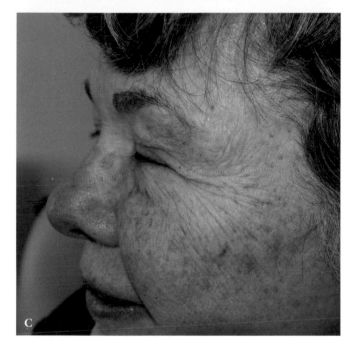

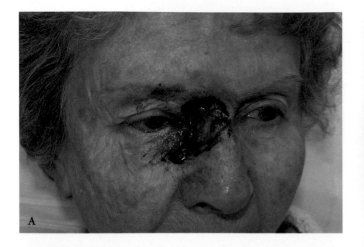

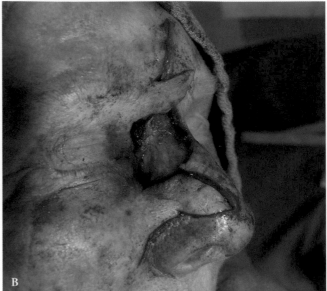

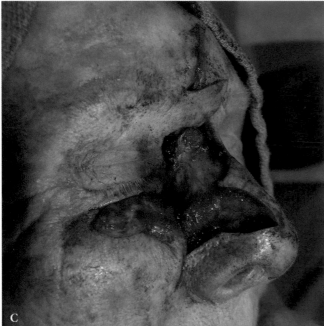

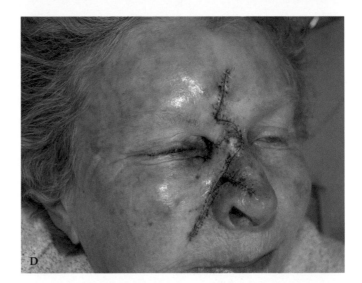

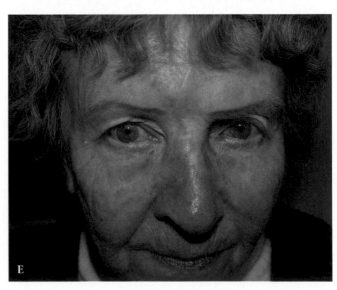

Figure 8.9 Bilateral Rhombic Transposition Flaps of Medial Canthus.

A. Complex defect involving the medial canthus, lower eyelid, and nasal sidewall. **B.** The superior rhombic flap is designed from the loose glabellar skin and the inferior rhombic flap is designed from the nasal sidewall skin. **C.** Both flaps lifted. **D.** Immediate post-op. Note that the medial canthus portion is left to heal by second intent, which is optimal in recreating a concave surface. **E.** Three months post-op.

CHAPTER 9

EAR RECONSTRUCTION

The three-dimensional nature of the ear with its many curves, peaks, and valleys demands the utmost attention to detail. Yet as challenging as it may seem, reconstruction of the ear can be made easier and predictable if one understands the surgical principles and anatomy.

The external ear is composed of skin and cartilage with the supporting nerves and blood vessels. The auricular cartilage provides a framework for all but the lobule of the ear. The tightly adherent skin extending from the preauricular sulcus to the helix produces distinct topographical landmarks that are important in understanding and describing the anterior ear.

Flaps, grafts, and primary linear closures can all be used in reconstruction of the ear. Healing by second intention is also a valuable tool. Deciding which reconstruction technique is best suited for a given defect depends upon its size and location. The goal is to restore the shape, size, and alignment of the ear. An important principle in ear reconstruction is that the entire anterior surface of both ears cannot be viewed simultaneously. It is therefore important to reconstruct the ear so that it is not distorted or deformed, but it need not exactly match the contralateral ear in size and appearance. The ear also has a functional importance for many patients as a supporting structure for eyeglasses.

The techniques covered in this chapter mainly address the repair of the helix, as the appearance of the ear is most profoundly affected by the shape and integrity of this structure.

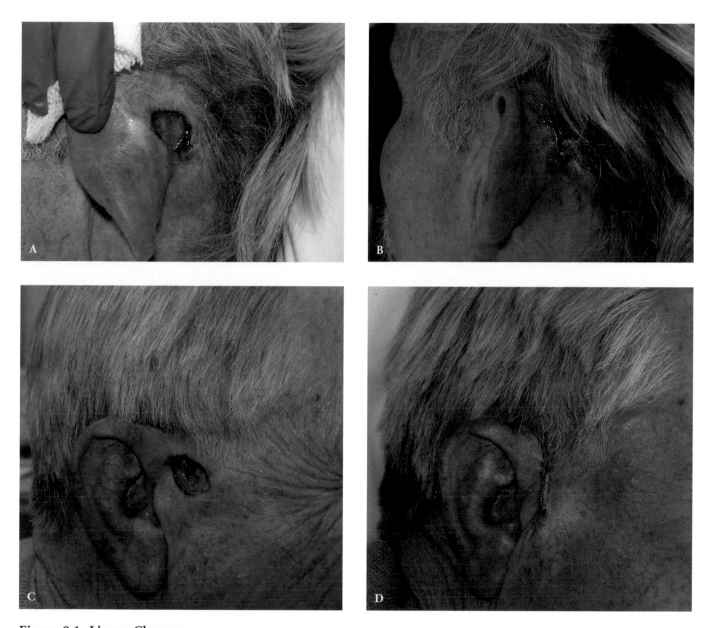

Figure 9.1 Linear Closure.

A–D. Defects on the pre- and postauricular creases can be closed primarily.

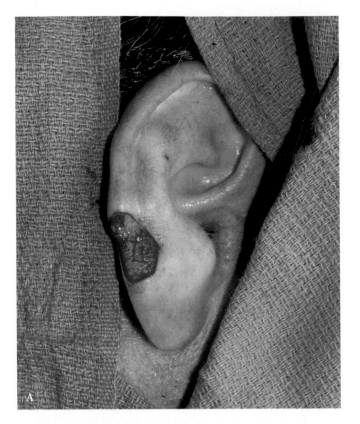

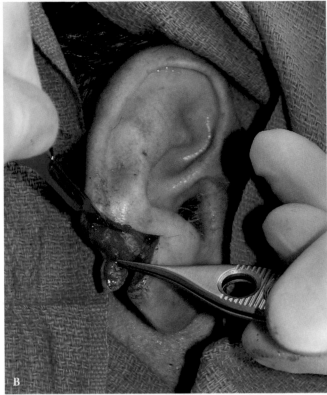

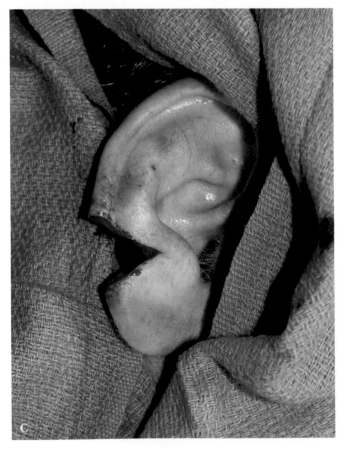

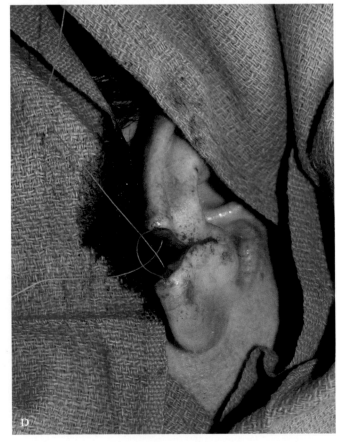

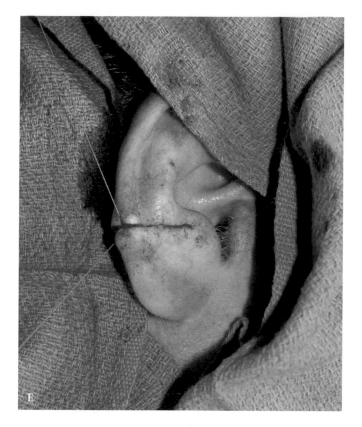

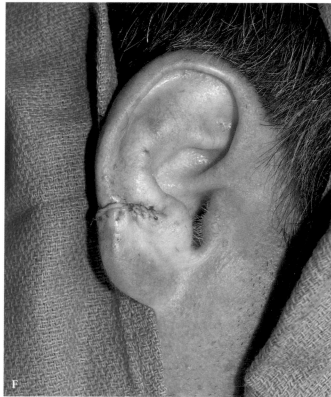

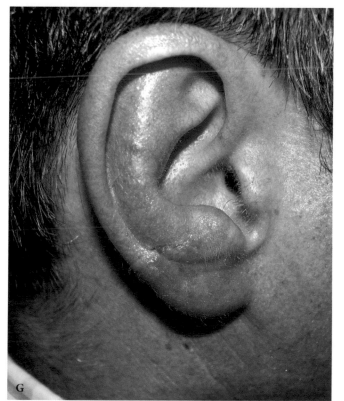

Figure 9.2 Wedge Excision Repair. Defects on most aspects of the helix can be repaired with a wedge excision repair as long as they are not large (typically, less than 1.5 cm).

A. Defect on the lower-mid helix. **B.** The principle behind the wedge closure is the conversion of the defect into a full-thickness (anterior skin, cartilage, posterior skin) triangular wedge. **C.** Ideally, the inner corner of the wedge is 30° in order to minimize the formation of a dog-ear. For larger defects, full thickness Burow's triangles can be excised superiorly and inferiorly to form a "star" to prevent excessive "cupping." **D, E.** The wedge is repaired by carefully reapproximating each layer: posterior skin, cartilage, and anterior skin. The helix must be realigned meticulously to prevent notching. Note the orientation of the buried suture at the helix, designed to maximally evert the helical rim. **F.** Use of vertical mattress sutures on the helix hclps prevent notching as well. **G.** Suture removal post-op.

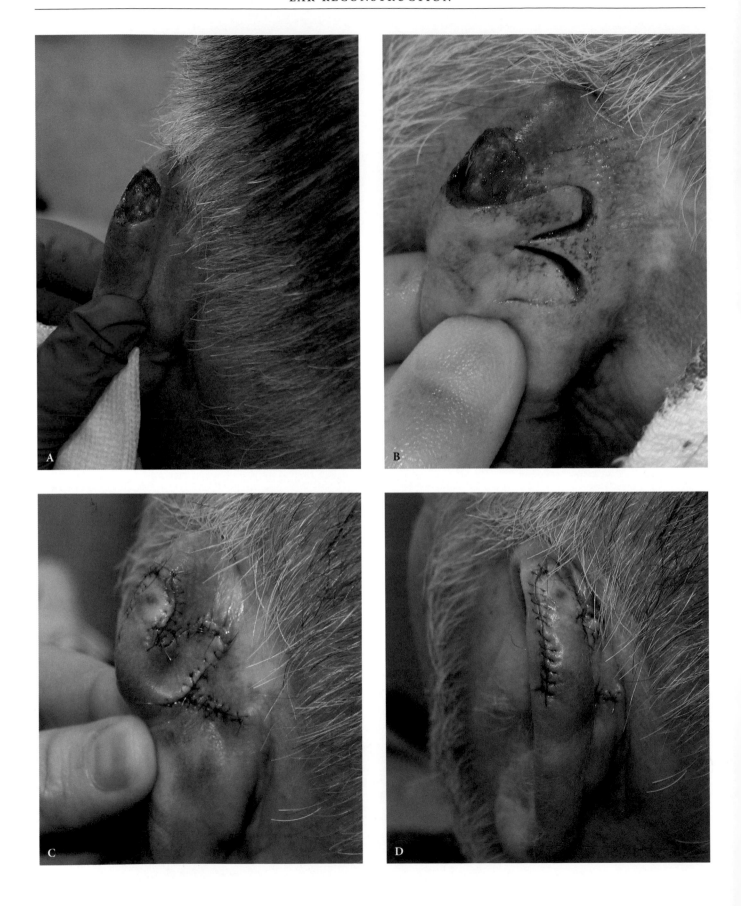

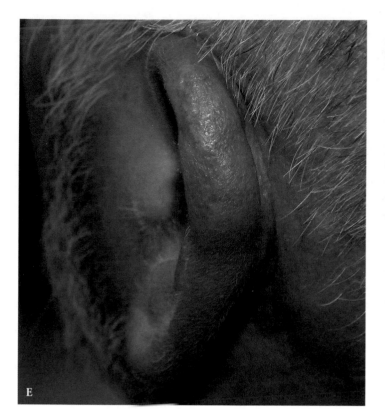
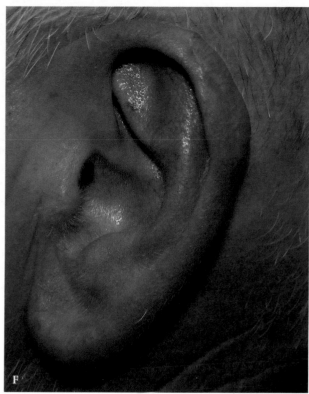

Figure 9.3 Bilobe Flap. Medium-sized defects on the superior and mid helix can also be repaired with the bilobe flap. Ideally, the cartilage should be intact, but there is enough bulk in the flap that it can offset a small cartilage defect.

A. Defect on the upper third of the helix with cartilage intact. **B.** Incisions are made with the total angle between the defect and the secondary lobe being approximately 90°. The loose postauricular skin is easily undermined in order to mobilize the flap. **C, D.** Immediate post-op. As with many ear repairs, there may be some initial distortion as the skin is stretched over the intact cartilage. This settles down rather quickly. **E, F.** Long-term post-op. Pincushioning is a common problem seen in bilobe flaps. This "problem" actually helps to reform the curvature and bulk of the helix.

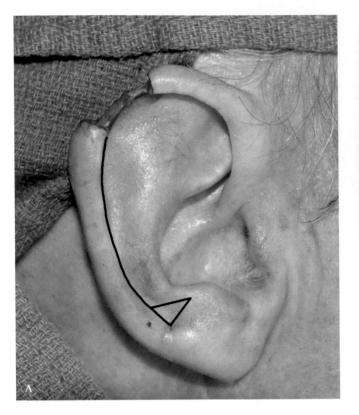

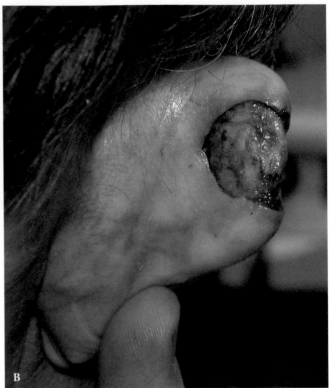

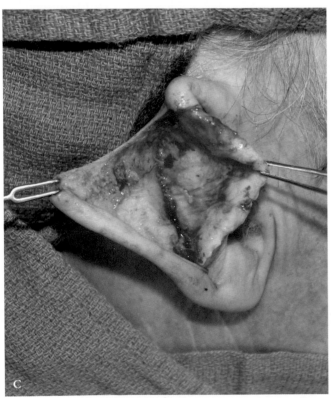

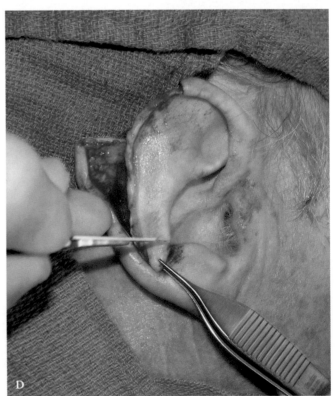

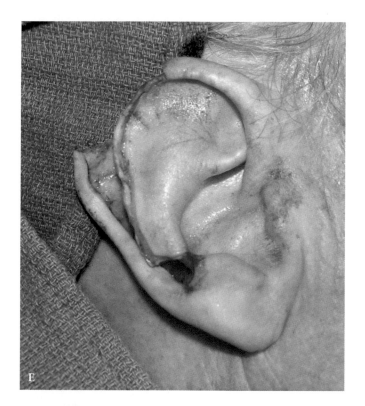

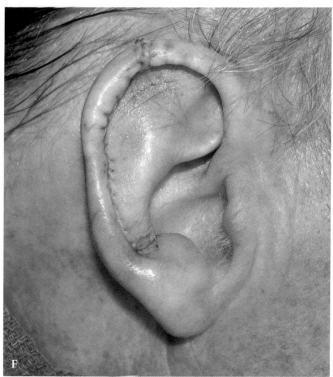

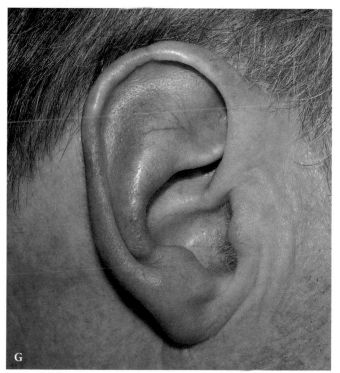

Figure 9.4 Chondrocutaneous Advancement Flap – Intact Cartilage. Defects confined to the helix less than 2.5 cm with or without a cartilage defect can be repaired with the chondrocutaneous advancement flap. There are two variations of the flap. It can be full-thickness and detached on both the anterior and posterior surfaces of the helix. This allows for maximal extension of the flap, although the flap pedicle is relatively narrow. The flap may also be designed with the posterior skin intact, leaving a broader flap base (as originally described by Antia and Buch).

A, B. Defect on the upper helix with the cartilage intact. Incision line is drawn, extending inferiorly. (For even greater movement, the incision can be made superiorly for a bilateral advancement.) **C.** The entire posterior skin is undermined at the level of the perichondrium in order to elevate the flap. **D, E.** A Burow's triangle is removed inferiorly to facilitate the release of the flap. **F.** The flap is then advanced superiorly with a dog-ear removed posteriorly. The helix needs to be realigned meticulously. **G.** One year post-op.

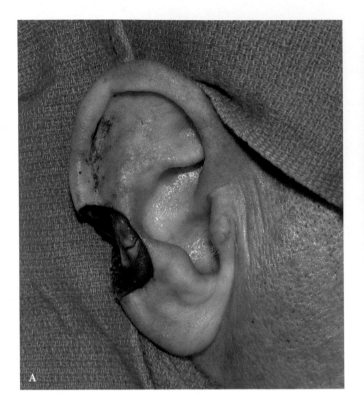

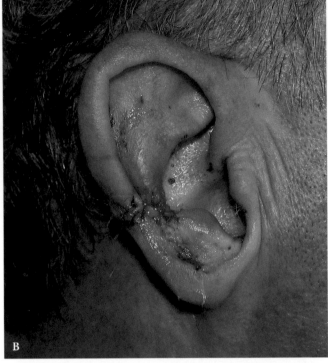

Figure 9.5 Chrondrocutaneous Advancement Flap – Missing Cartilage.

A. Defect with helical cartilage involvement. The helical flap includes a small strip of cartilage, as this allows for a better replacement of the missing cartilage in the defect. **B.** Immediate post-op. Burow's triangle removed from the lobule. **D.** Six-week post-op.

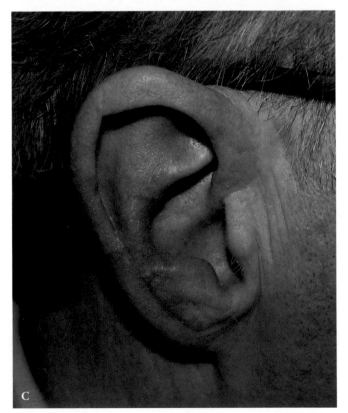

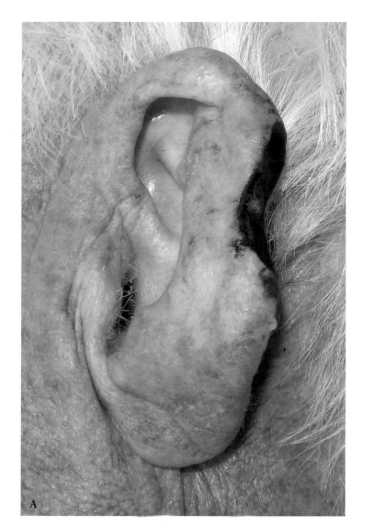

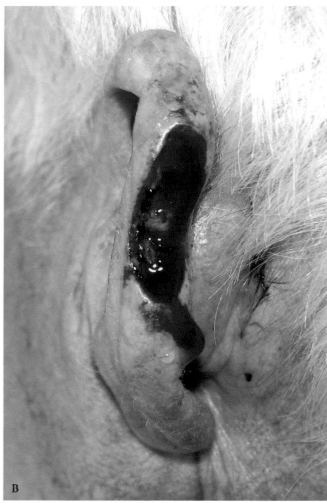

Figure 9.6 Bilateral Island Pedicle Flap. The bilateral island pedicle flap can be used for longer defects on the rim in place a two-stage pedicle flap.

A, B. Long defect on the helical rim. **C.** Island pedicle flaps advanced from superior and inferior directions. **D.** Immediate post-op. **E.** Six-week post-op. The island pedicle flap has a tendency to pincushion, which in this case helps to recreate the contour of the helix.

(Continued on next page.)

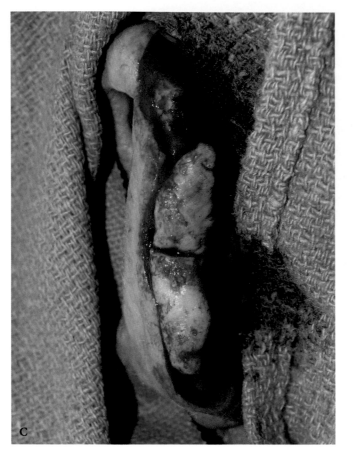

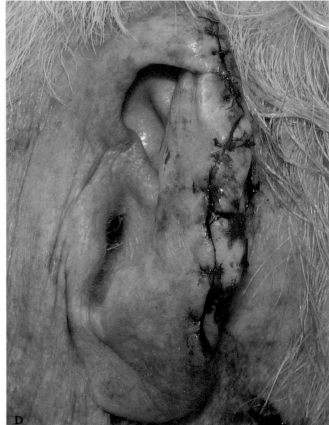

Figure 9.6 Bilateral Island Pedicle Flap *(continued)*.

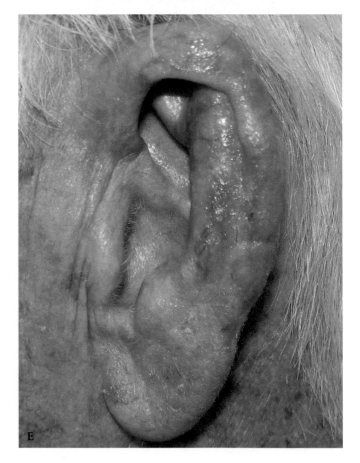

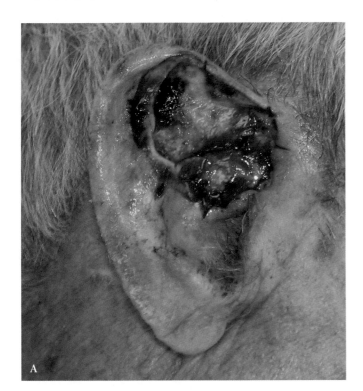

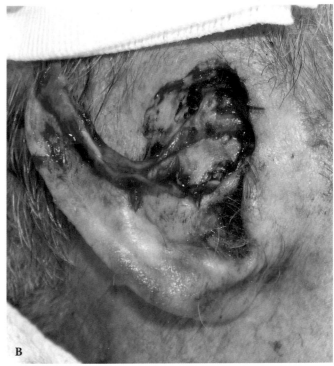

Figure 9.7 Wedge Repair and Full-Thickness Skin Graft. Complex defects can be repaired by combining different reconstructive techniques.

A. Defect with substantial loss of cartilage and thinning of helical rim superiorly. **B.** The posterior ear skin and the thinned aspect of the rim are excised and used as a full-thickness skin graft. **C.** The exposed helical rim is advanced and attached near the helical root to reform the helix. **D.** A full-thickness skin graft is applied to the central defect to prevent buckling. **E.** Two-month post-op. **F.** Comparison with the contralateral ear.

(Continued on next page.)

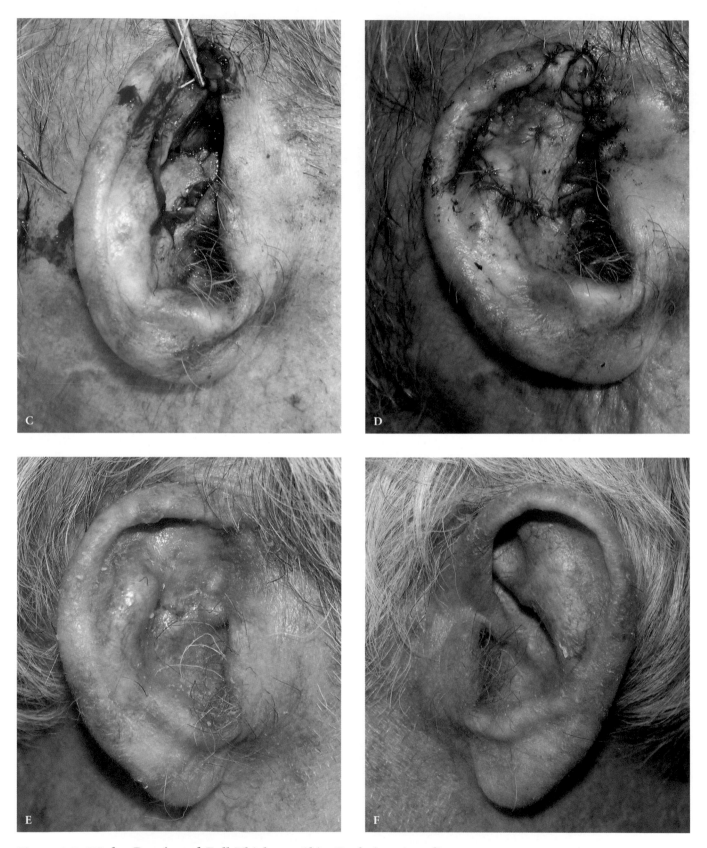

Figure 9.7 Wedge Repair and Full-Thickness Skin Graft *(continued).*

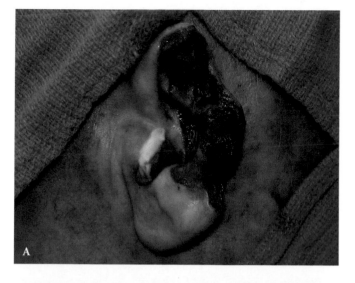

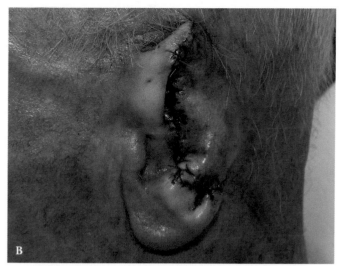

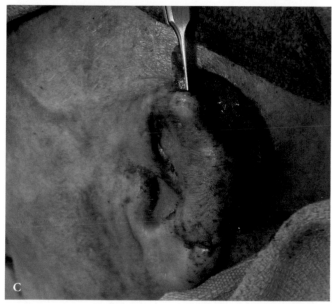

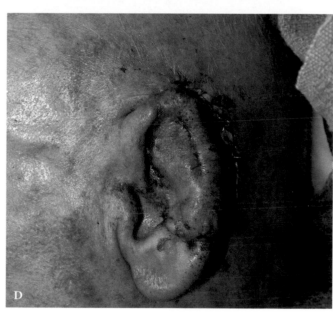

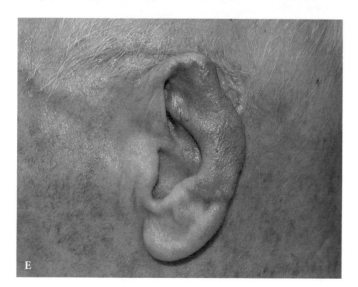

Figure 9.8 Retroauricular Staged Pedicle Flap. Full-thickness defects with significant loss of width and height may require this two-stage procedure

A. Defect involving the helix and antehelix. Incisions made from the defect extending posteriorly. Flap is raised from the posterior ear and postauricular skin. **B.** Flap draped and sutured into position. **C.** Detachment at 3 weeks with insertion of cartilage obtained from postauricular sulcus. **D.** Immediate post-op. Split-thickness skin graft applied to the postauricular skin. **E.** Two-month follow-up.

(Continued on next page.)

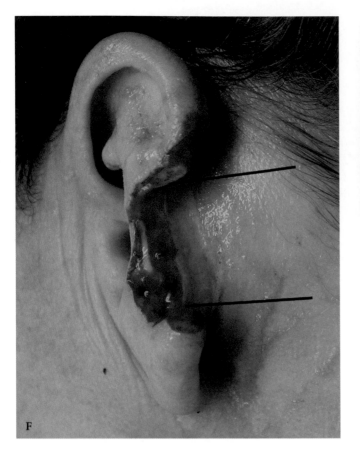

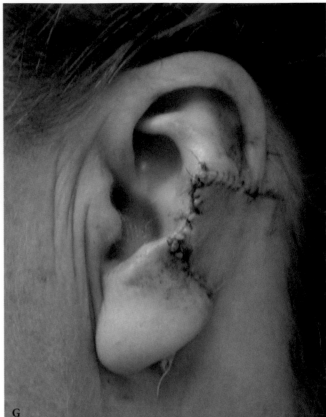

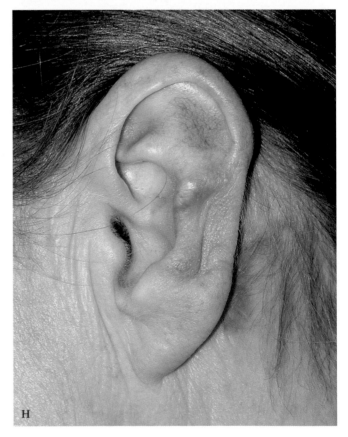

Figure 9.8 Retroauricular Staged Pedicle Flap (*continued*).

F. Full-thickness defect with flap incisions drawn.
G. Postauricular flap draped and sutured into place.
H. Two months post detachment prior to any revision surgery.

CHAPTER 10

NOSE

Reconstruction of the nose can be very challenging because of its central prominence and the need for precise symmetry. The topography of the nose is quite unique, with its three-dimensional contours and the subtle convex and concave surfaces. A thorough understanding of the anatomy is vital, prior to surgery.

The framework of the nose is comprised of the nasal bone, two upper lateral cartilages, and the two lower lateral (alar) cartilages. The inner aspect is lined with mucosa, and the outer aspect is covered with muscle, fibrous tissue, and skin. Although most defects on the nose encompass the skin only, the reconstruction may also entail manipulating cartilage, mucosa, and muscle.

The skin of the nose can be divided by its morphologic appearance into thirds. The lower third is more sebaceous, while the upper two thirds have a smoother consistency. Matching these traits is important for the best cosmetic outcome.

The nose is further divided into many cosmetic subunits and junctions. Respecting and recreating these subunits is critical.

Lastly, one must not forget the functional aspect of the nose. Care must be taken to preserve or recreate the internal and external valves.

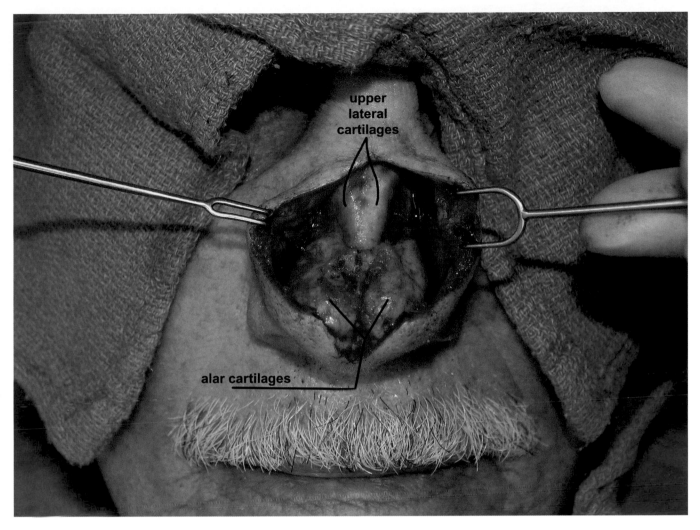

Figure 10.1 Anatomy.

Nasal cartilages – upper lateral and lower lateral (alar) cartilages.

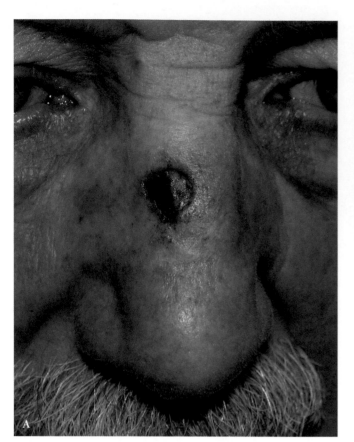

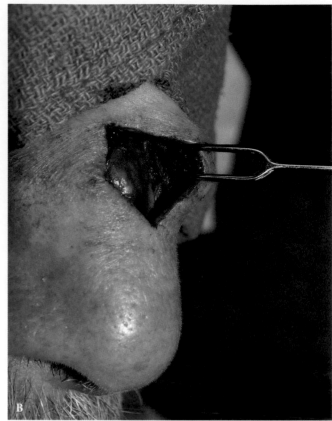

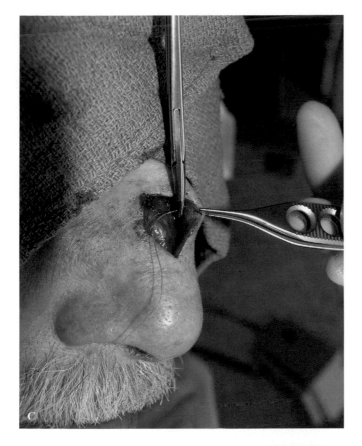

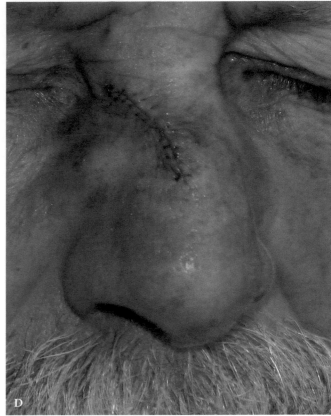

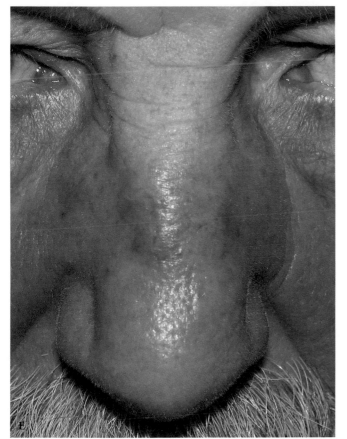

Figure 10.2 Linear Closure. Many small- to medium-size defects can be closed primarily on the nasal dorsum and tip.

A. Defect on dorsum. **B.** The muscle base of the defect is removed to expose perichondrium or periosteum and dog-ears are removed superiorly and inferiorly along the relaxed skin tension lines. The wound is widely undermined in the submuscular plane. **C.** The wound edges are reapproximated with sutures grasping the muscle so that there is minimal tension on the overlying skin. **D.** Immediate post-op. Note the wound eversion. **E.** One month post-op.

(Continued on next page.)

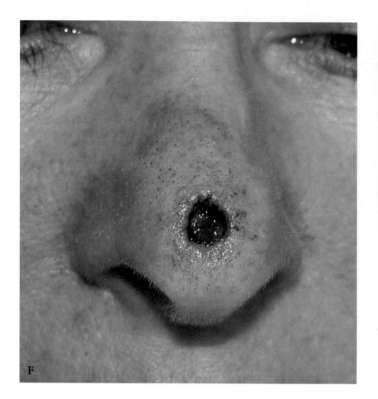

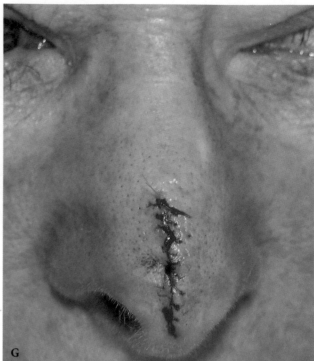

Figure 10.2 Linear Closure *(continued).*

F. Small defects on the nasal tip can also be closed primarily. Undermining is done in the same plane and the fascia/muscle reapproximated. **G.** Immediate post-op. The length of the incision is longer than 3:1 in order to taper the ends over the curvature of the nasal tip. Note the good wound eversion, which resulted from the reapproximation of the muscle fascia layer. **H.** Three months post-op. Note that the distortion seen in immediate post-op has been resolved.

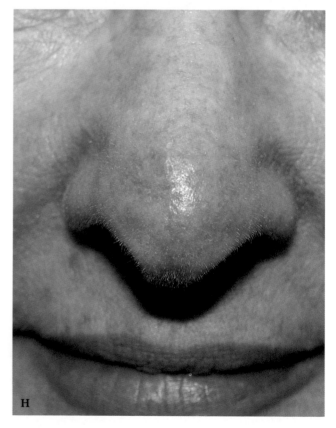

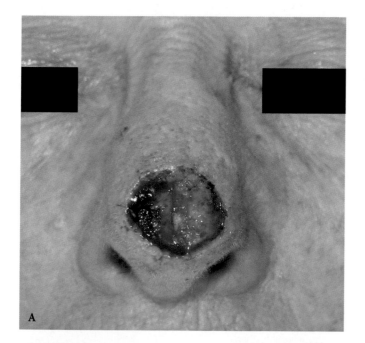

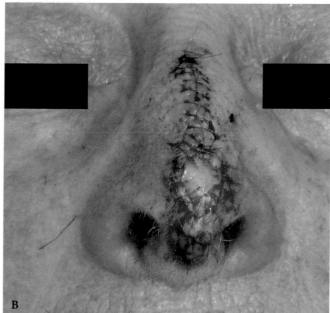

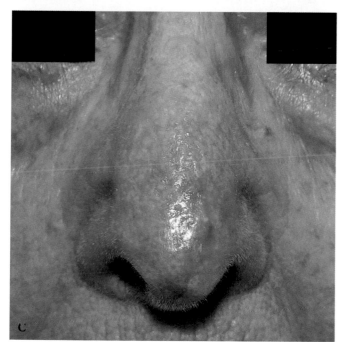

Figure 10.3 Burow's Graft. Medium-size nasal tip defects can be repaired with a Burow's graft, which provides the best skin graft match.

A. Defect on the nasal tip. Burow's graft is obtained from the superior dog-ear. **B.** Immediate post-op. A small inferior dog-ear is also taken so that the defect is in the shape of a fusiform ellipse. Both the superior and inferior portions of the defect are then partially closed to yield a central defect that is smaller than the original. **C.** Two months post-op. Note that the distortion is resolved.

(Continued on next page.)

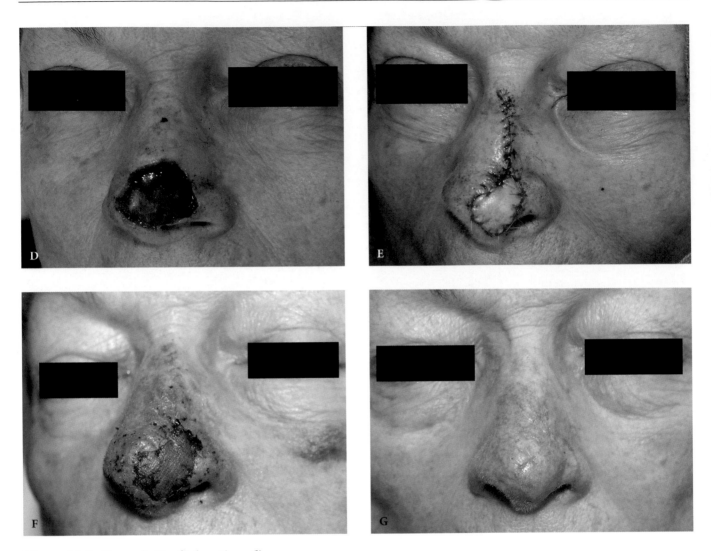

Figure 10.3 Burow's Graft *(continued).*

D. Sometimes larger defects can be closed with a Burow's graft. **E.** Immediate post-op. **F.** One week post-op. The dusky color of the graft does not necessarily portend poor outcome. **G.** Two months post-op.

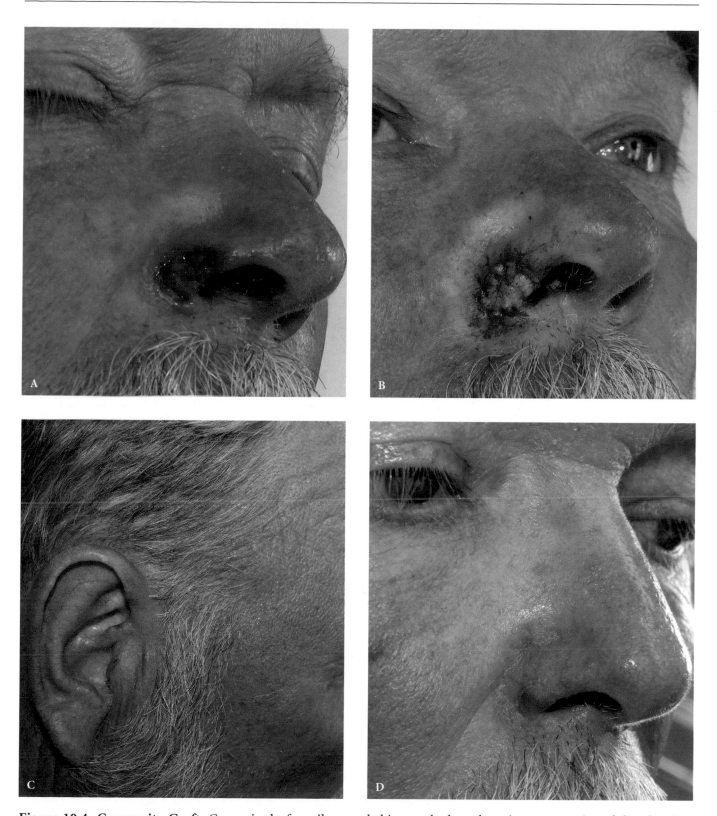

Figure 10.4 Composite Graft. Comprised of cartilage and skin, used when there is compromise of the alar rim.

A. Defect on the nasal alar rim. **B.** Immediate post-op of composite graft taken from the anterior helical rim of the ear (refer to Chapter 4 for detailed information on harvesting a composite graft). **C.** Two months post-op. **D.** Two months post-op of donor site.

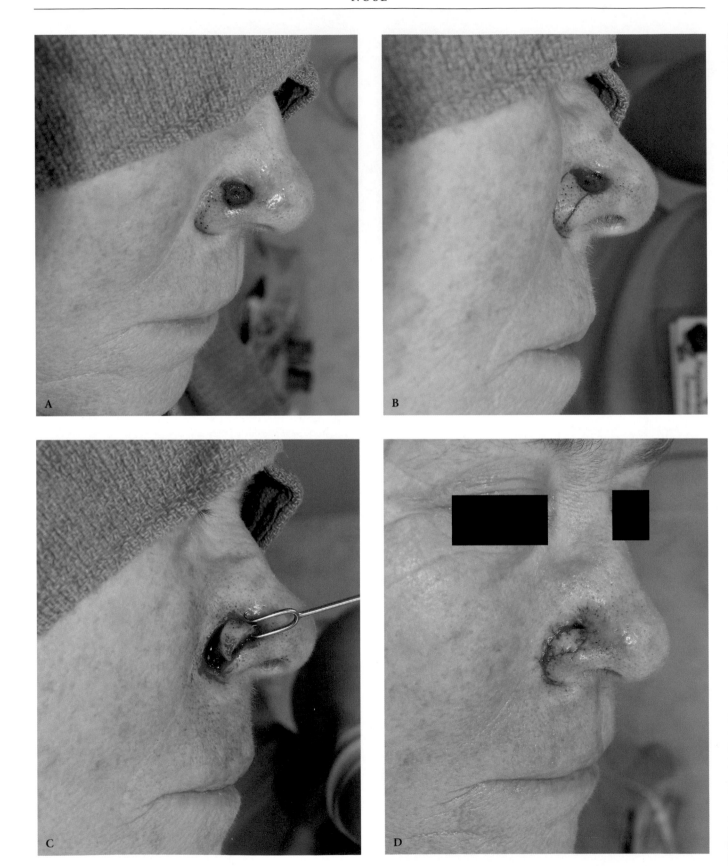

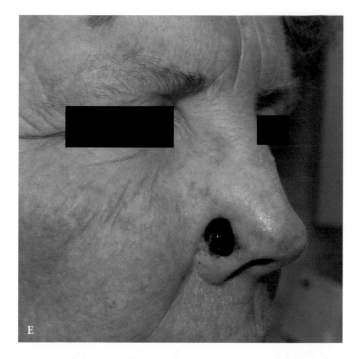

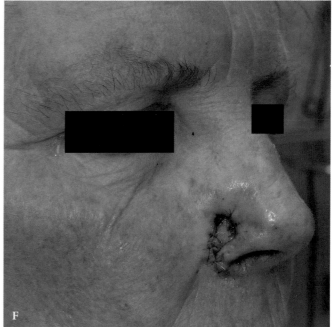

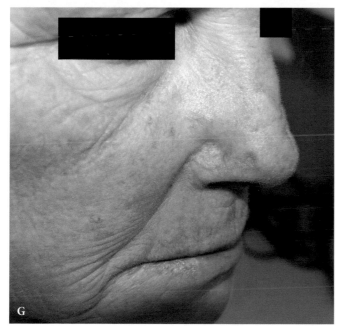

Figure 10.5 Island Pedicle Flap – Nasal Ala.

A. Defect on the nasal ala. **B.** Island pedicle flap is designed so that the body of the flap is long and does not taper until it reaches the inferior portion of the lateral ala. This prevents retraction of the ala when the secondary defect is closed. **C.** The flap is mobilized after careful undermining of the pedicle. **D.** Immediate post-op. Note the lack of retraction of the alar rim. **E.** Defect on the alar rim involving the crease. **F.** Immediate post-op. The superior portion is allowed to heal by second intent to recreate the crease. **G.** One year post-op.

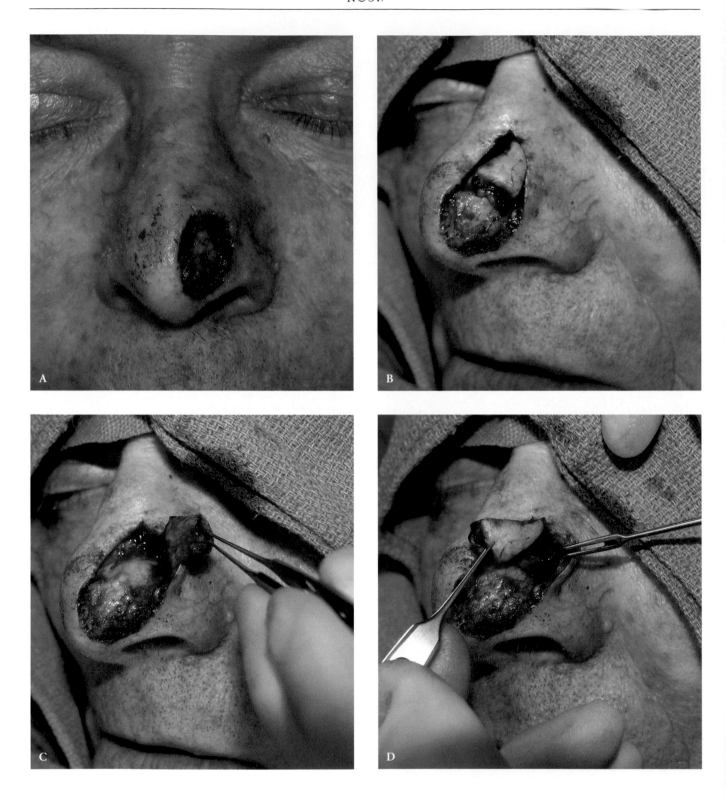

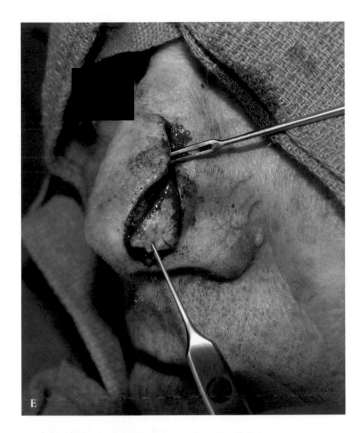

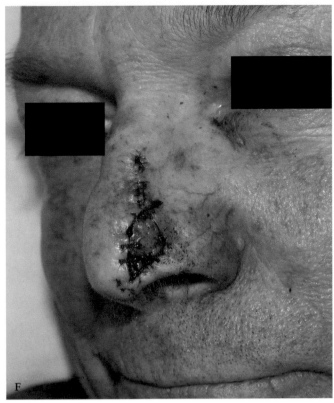

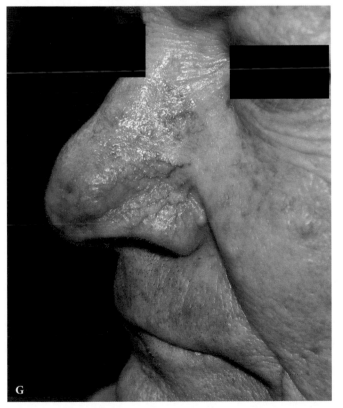

Figure 10.6 Single Sling Island Pedicle Flap of Papadopolous.

A. Defect on the lateral nasal tip. **B.** Island pedicle flap designed superiorly. This variation is unique in that the muscular pedicle is either medial or lateral to the flap instead of deep to the flap. **C.** The nasalis muscle is isolated using bi-level undermining – below the nasalis muscle **D.** and above the nasalis muscle. **E.** The flap rotates on the single sling of nasalis muscle far greater than the traditional island pedicle flap. **F.** Immediate post-op. **G.** One month post-op.

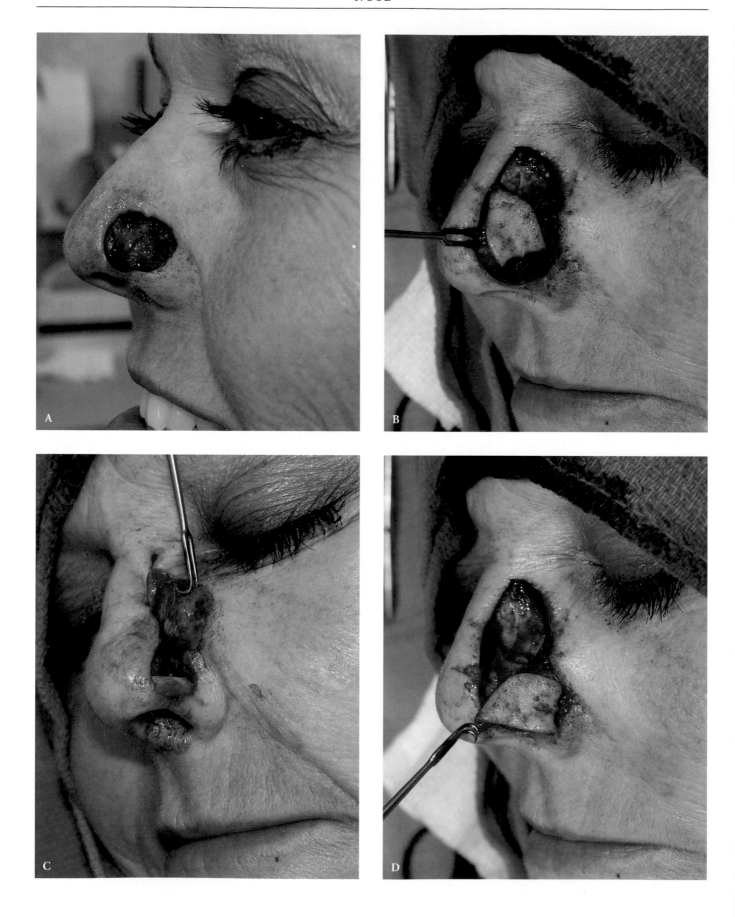

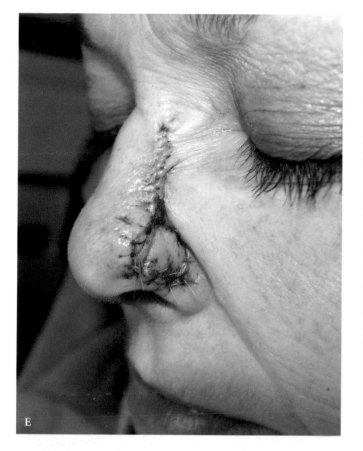

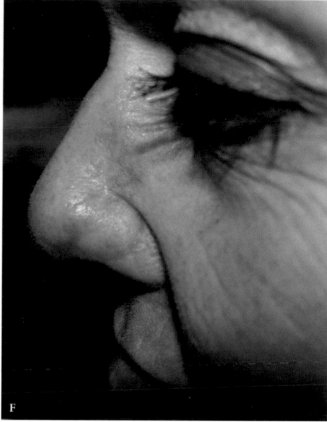

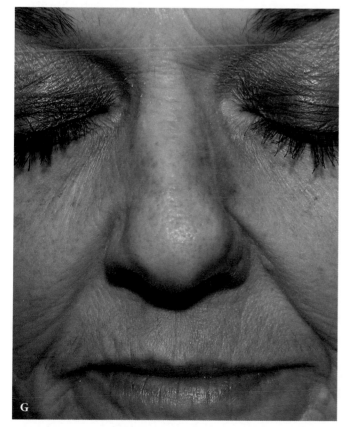

Figure 10.7 Single Sling Island Pedicle flap with Cartilage Graft.

A. Defect on the distal lateral nasal tip and alar rim. **B.** Muscular sling is mobilized laterally. **C.** Cartilage graft harvested from the ear is used to support the alar rim. **D.** The flap is rotated 90° to better fit the horizontally shaped defect. **E.** Immediate post-op. **F,G.** Three months post-op.

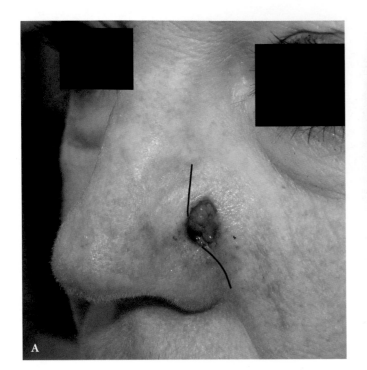

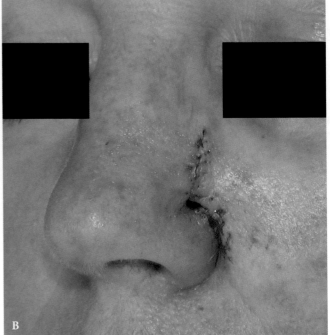

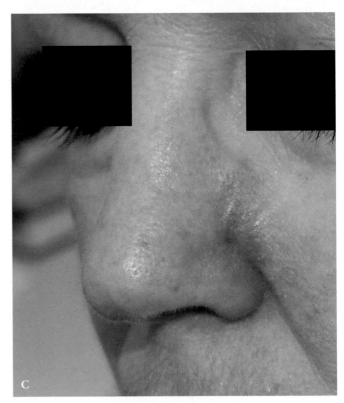

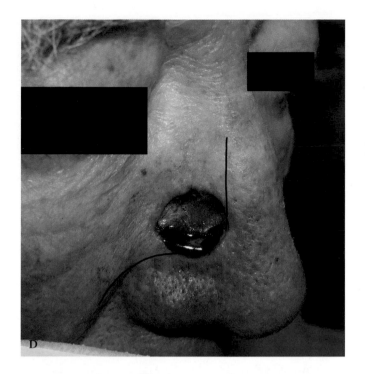

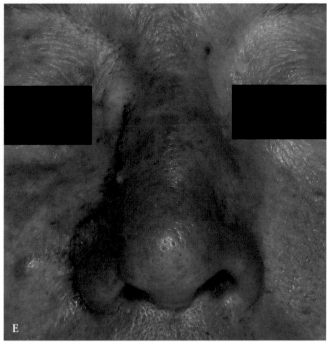

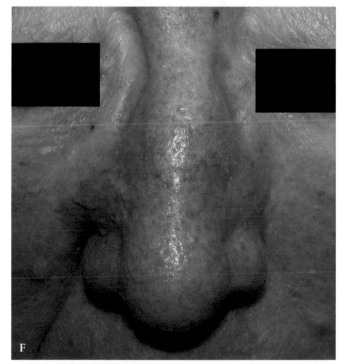

Figure 10.8 Crescentic Advancement Flap.

A. Defect on the nasal sidewall near the alar crease. **B.** Immediate post-op. Incision follows the alar crease inferiorly and a small dog-ear is removed superiorly. **C.** One month post-op. **D.** Larger defect on the nasal sidewall. **E.** Immediate post-op. **F.** Six weeks post-op.

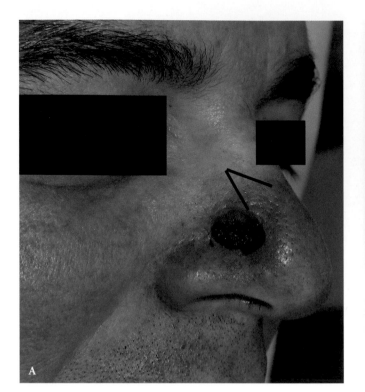

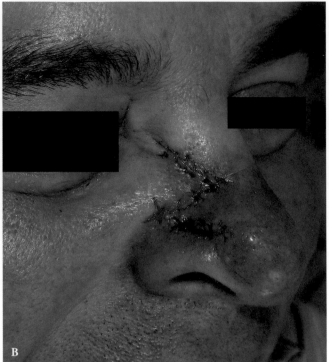

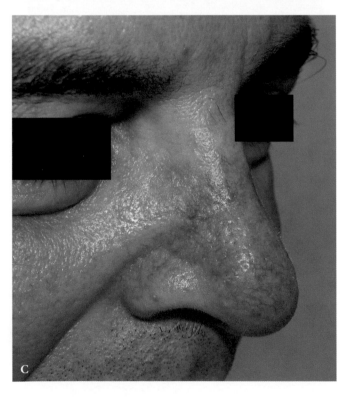

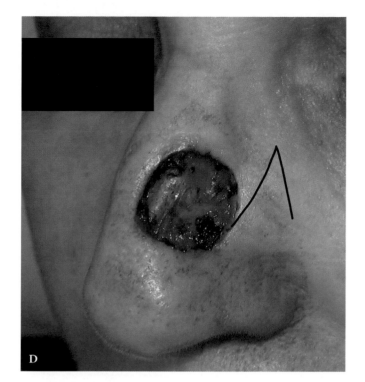

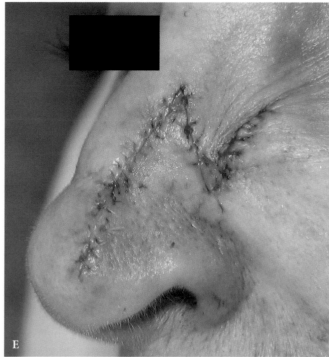

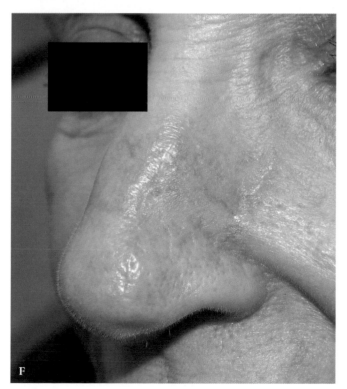

Figure 10.9 Rhombic Transposition Flap. Defects on the supratip, dorsum, and sidewall are amenable to repair with rhombic flap.

A. Defect on the lateral supratip. **B.** Immediate post-op. Superiorly based rhombic transposition flap. **C.** Two months post-op **D.** Defect on the nasal dorsum and sidewall. **E.** Immediate post-op. Laterally based rhombic transposition flap. **F.** Two months post-op.

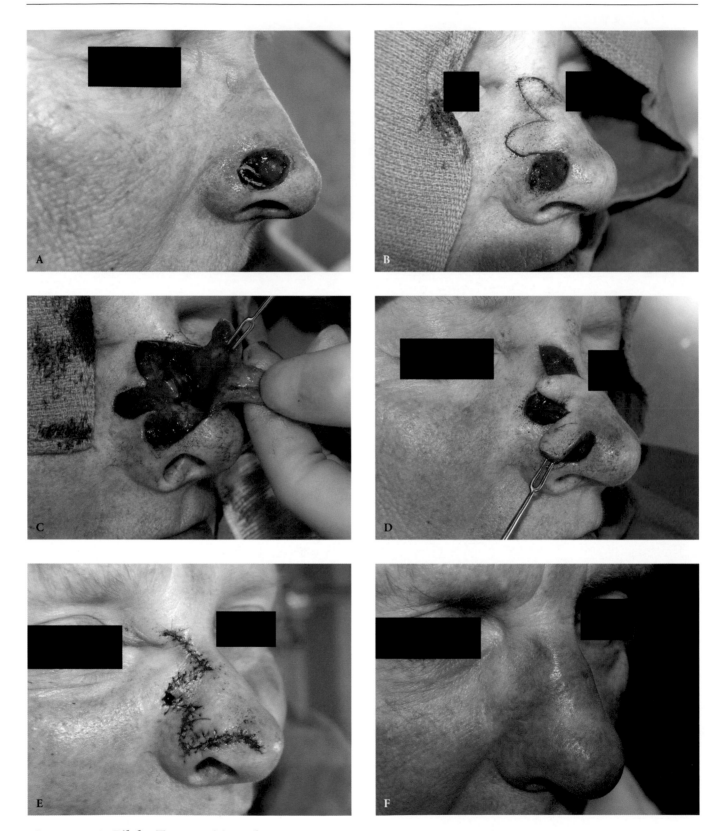

Figure 10.10 Bilobe Transposition Flap.

A. Defect on the lateral tip. **B.** Bilobe flap based medially. **C.** Flap undermined in the submuscular plane. **D.** Flap movement. **E.** Immediate post-op. **F.** One year post-op.

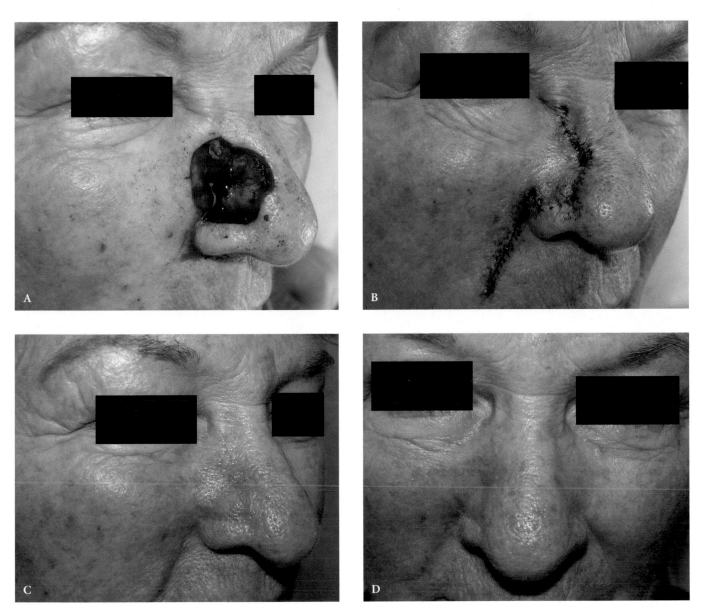

Figure 10.11 Nasolabial Transposition Flap.

A. Large defect on the nasal sidewall and ala. **B.** Immediate post-op. Transposition flap designed from the nasolabial fold and draped into place. Note the extreme concavity of the flap that has resulted from a periosteal tacking suture. **C, D.** Three months post-op. Note the symmetry that has resulted from the tacking suture.

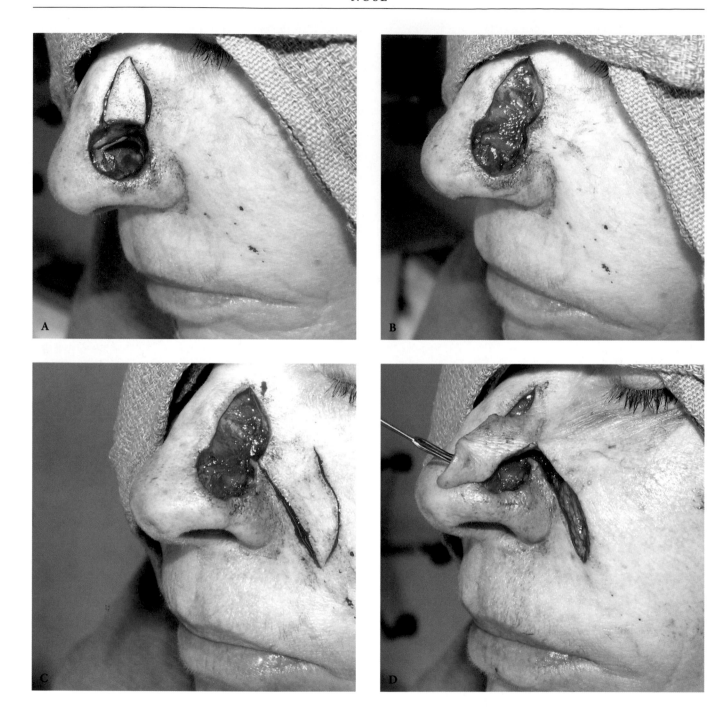

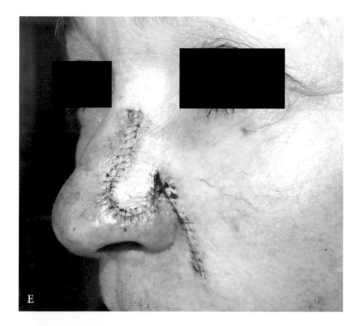

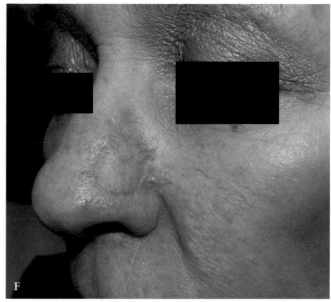

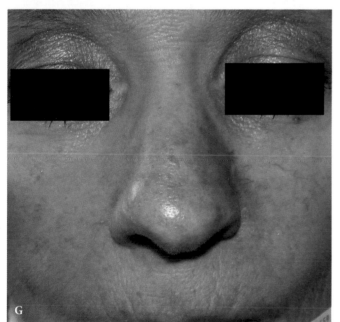

Figure 10.12 Nasolabial Transposition Flap Combined with Hinged Flap.

A. Through-and-through defect on the nasal sidewall and ala. Hinged flap designed superiorly (similar to an island pedicle flap). **B.** The flap is hinged downward (like opening a book) to resurface the inner lining of the defect. **C.** Nasolabial transposition flap incised. **D.** Flap is lifted and transposed to cover the anterior aspect of the defect. **E.** Immediate post-op **F.** One month post-op. **G.** Two month post-op. Note the symmetry.

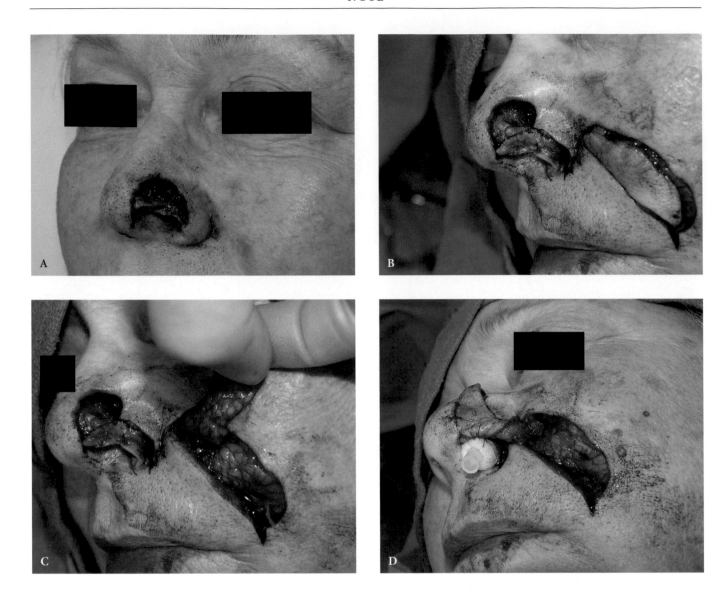

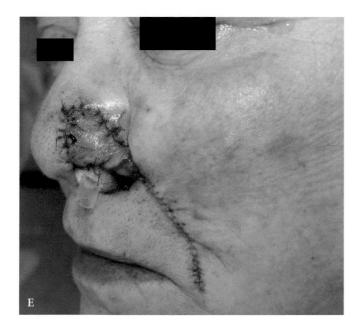

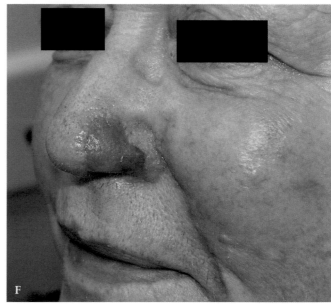

Figure 10.13 Hinged and Interpolated Flaps.

A. Defect involving nasal tip, sidewall, ala with full thickness defect of the alar rim. **B.** The remaining ala is lifted and turned inward on a hinge (like opening a book) and secured to resurface the inner aspect of the full thickness portion of the defect. (This is similar to an island pedicle flap.) Nasolabial interpolated flap is designed laterally. **C.** The interpolated flap is dissected until the only attachment is the muscular pedicle. **D.** The flap is draped to resurface the anterior portion of the defect. **E.** Immediate post-op. The flap is attached by the muscular pedicle for three weeks and then detached. **F.** One week post detachment.

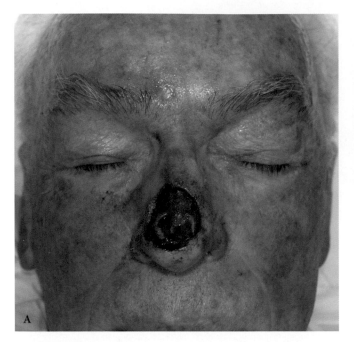

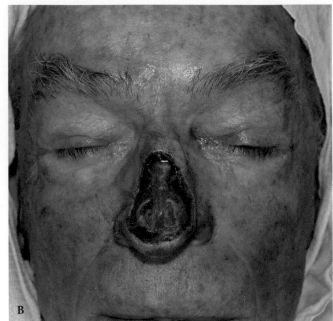

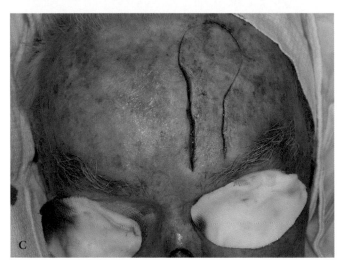

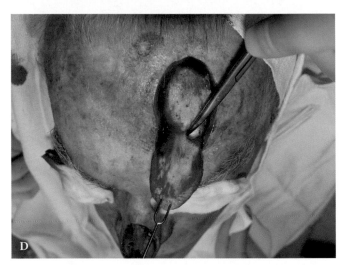

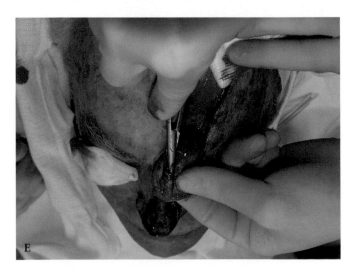

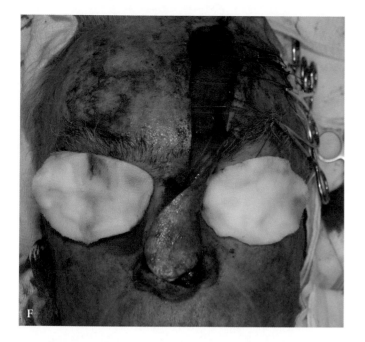

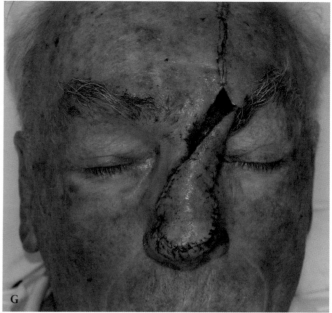

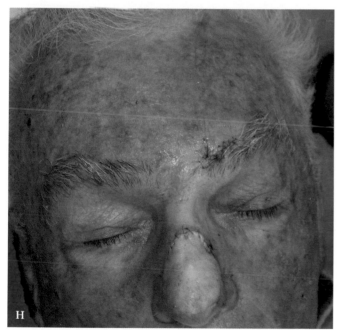

Figure 10.14 Paramedian Forehead Flap.

A. Large defect on the nasal dorsum and tip. **B.** The defect is extended superiorly and inferiorly to encompass the cosmetic subunits. **C.** The flap is based on the supratrochlear artery. Incision made along the artery and around the templated area. **D.** Flap is undermined below the frontalis muscle on the periosteum. **E.** The distal portion of the flap is stripped of the frontalis muscle. **F.** The flap is draped into place, and the donor site is sutured. **G.** Immediate post-op. **H.** Detachment at three weeks. The pedicle is severed, and the proximal aspect of the flap is inset.

(Continued on next page.)

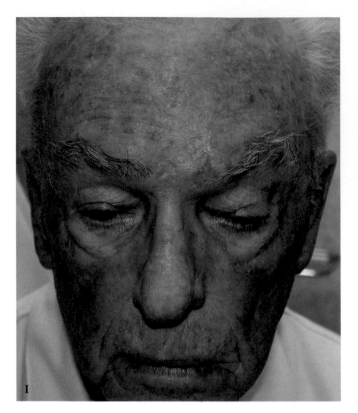

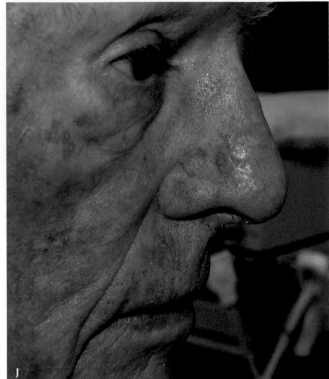

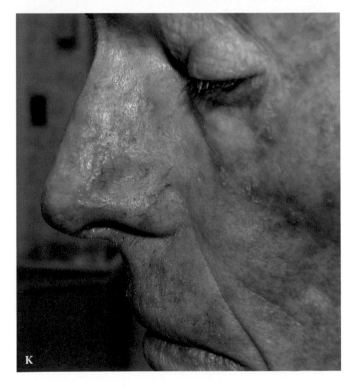

Figure 10.14 Paramedian Forehead Flap *(continued).*

I–K. Two months post-op.

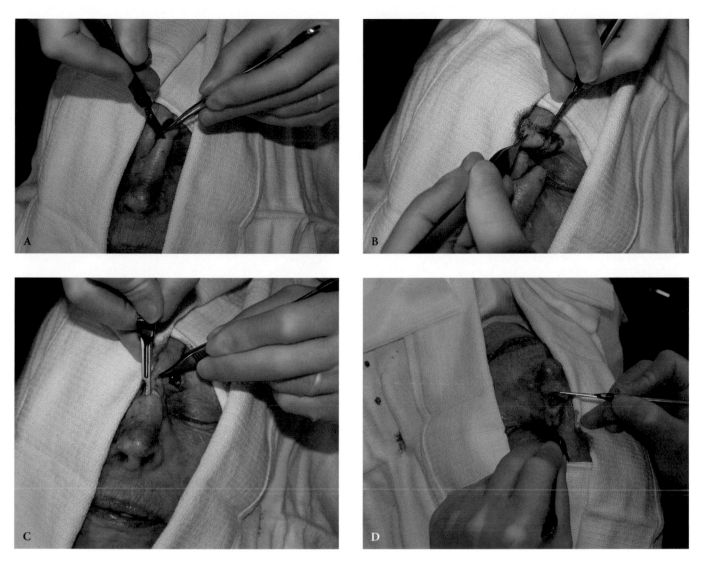

Figure 10.15 Paramedial Forehead Flap Takedown.

A. At approximately three weeks, the pedicle is bisected. **B.** The proximal stalk is excised. **C, D.** The flap is beveled, trimmed, debulked to fit the underlying defect.

(Continued on next page.)

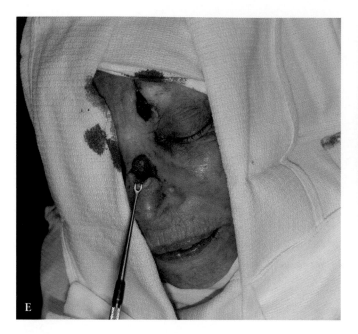
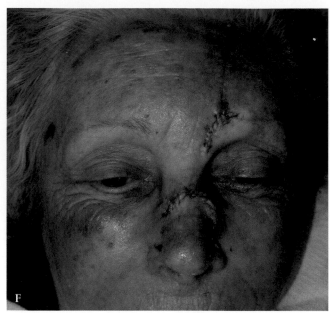

Figure 10.15 Paramedial Forehead Flap Takedown *(continued).*

E, F. The two ends are then sutured into place.

CHAPTER 11

LIPS AND CHIN

The lips are comprised of the upper and lower lips with both a vermilion and a cutaneous component. The lips are bordered by the melolabial folds laterally, the nose superiorly, and the mental crease inferiorly. The reconstruction of the lips involves meticulous attention to both the cosmetic and functional outcome.

The movement of the lips results from the underlying orbicularis oris muscle, which functions as a sphincter. Fortunately, significant portions of the muscle can be removed and function restored with careful reapproximation. The vascular supply to the lips is rich and well anastamosed. The labial arteries course through the orbicularis muscle on the posterior aspects of the vermilion lip.

Although there are many important reconstruction concepts in the cosmetic appearance of the lip, two simple ones stand out. First is the need for careful reapproximation of the vermilion border. Marking the borders prior to the anesthesia is important. The second is keeping all incisions in the cosmetic junctions or the relaxed skin tension lines. The cosmetic junctions are the vermilion borders, melolabial folds, nasolabial junction, and mental crease. The relaxed skin tension lines emanate vertically in the central lip and radiate in a slightly lateral direction at the commissures. These can be seen readily when one purses the lips. Horizontal lines on the cutaneous lips are very noticeable.

The chin is included with the lip because of its proximity. Most defects on the chin are repaired in a vertical direction, although it is difficult to precisely elicit the relaxed skin tension line. Additionally, the mental crease is an important junction to respect. Therefore, incisions in the chin should be either kept vertical or within the mental crease.

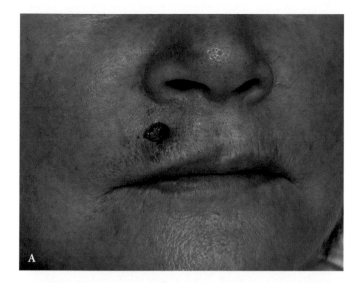

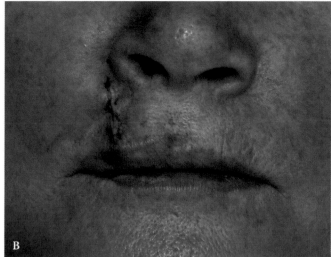

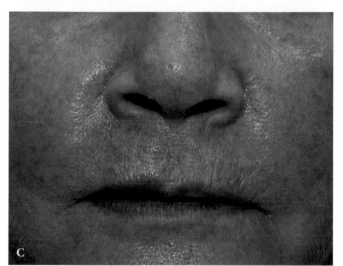

Figure 11.1 Linear Closure.

A. Defect on the upper cutaneous lip. **B.** Immediate post-op. Linear closure in the vertical direction, which is in the relaxed skin tension line, accentuated when the lip is pursed. The RSTL becomes more oblique laterally. The inferior aspect of the incision ends prior to the vermilion border, which is possible because the defect is high on the lip. In more inferior defects, it is permissible to extend the dog-ear through the vermilion border. Care must be taken to reapproximate the vermilion border. Note the extensive wound eversion, which is especially important in area with furrows. **C.** Two months post-op.

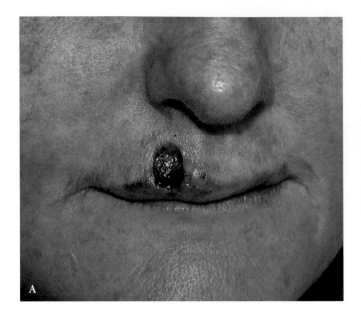

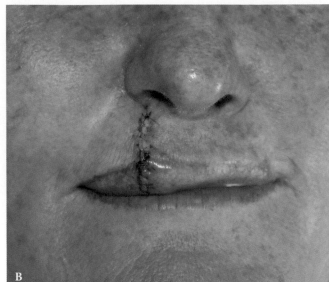

Figure 11.2 Linear Closure.

A. Defect involving both the upper cutaneous and vermilion lip. Note the preoperative markings of the vermilion border **B.** Immediate post-op. Small to medium defects of the upper cutaneous lip, close to or involving the vermilion, can simply be repaired primarily with a partial lip wedge of the inferior dog-ear. The incision should be carried through to the wet mucosa so that there is no protrusion of the vermilion. The muscle and muscosa are repaired in separate layers (see lip wedge). **C.** Two months post-op. Note the precise reapproximation of the vermilion border.

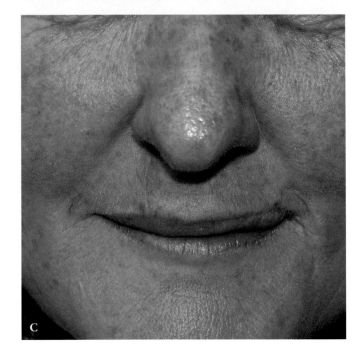

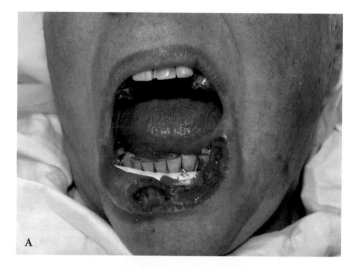

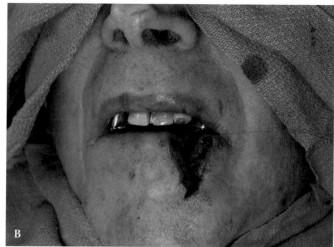

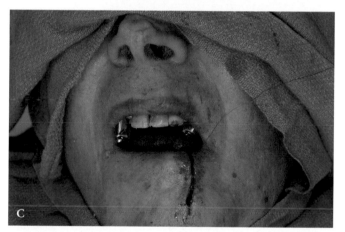

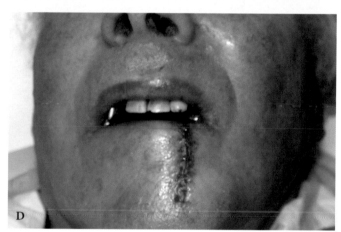

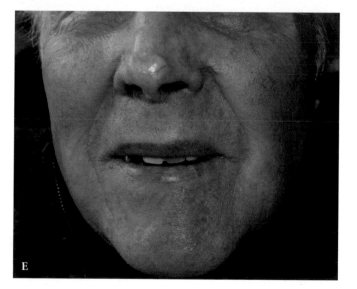

Figure 11.3 Lip Wedge Repair.

A. Full-thickness defect of the lower lip involving the skin, muscle, and mucosa. Wedge repair can be used for defects encompassing up to one third of the lip, although larger defects can sometimes be closed in this manner. **B.** A full-thickness V-excision is made inferiorly. An M-plasty can be used inferiorly to end the incision at the mental crease. The defect is closed sequentially from inferior to superior and posterior to anterior in layers. First the mucosa is repaired using a running 5–0 chromic suture. **C.** The orbicularis oris is reapproximated using with a series of interrupted sutures making sure that the vermilion borders match up precisely. The dermis is then reapproximated. **D.** The mucosal and skin sutures are sewn inferior to superior until they are tied off at the vermilion border. **E.** Nine months post-op.

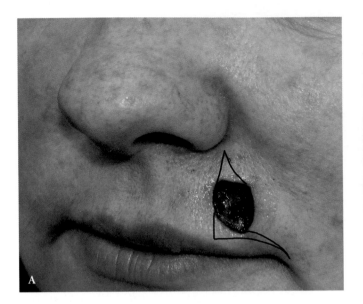

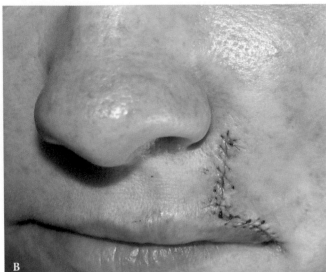

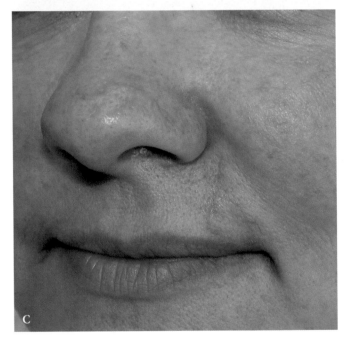

Figure 11.4 Advancement Flap – O-to-L Type.

A. Defect on the inferior aspect of the upper cutaneous lip. **B.** The flap incision is made along the vermilion border to the oral commissure and the dog-ear taken out superiorly along the RSTL. In larger defects, the incision can extended further laterally. **C.** Three weeks post-op. Note that the medial displacement of the melolabial fold has resolved.

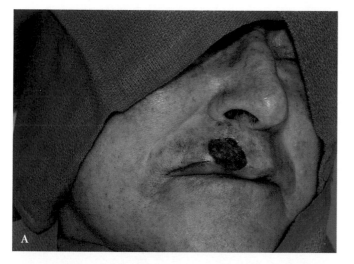

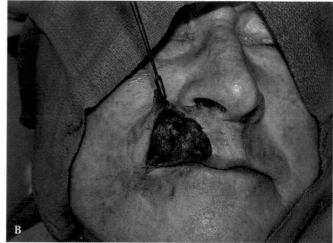

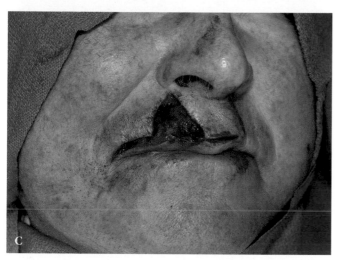

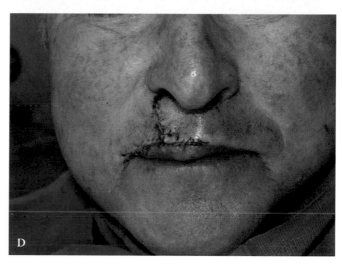

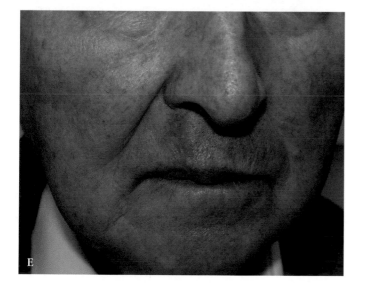

Figure 11.5 Advancement Flap – O-to-T Type.

A. Defect on the upper cutaneous and vermilion lip with underlying muscle intact. An incision is made laterally along the vemilion border. **B.** Flap is raised laterally to assess movement. **C.** Incision is made along the medial vermilion border to gain further mobility. **D.** Immediate post-op. The vermilion portion of the defect was advanced superiorly. **E.** Six weeks post-op.

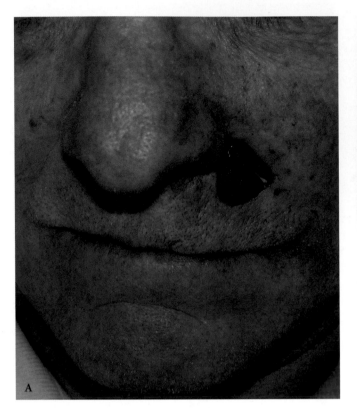

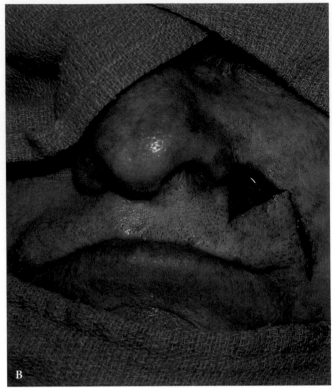

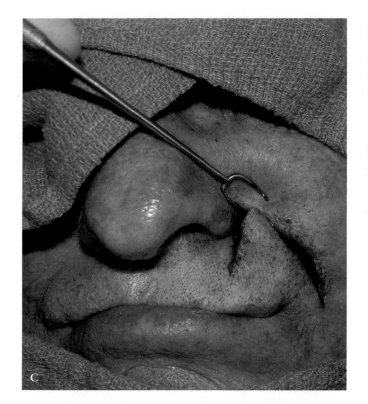

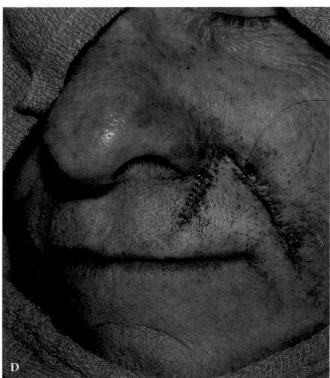

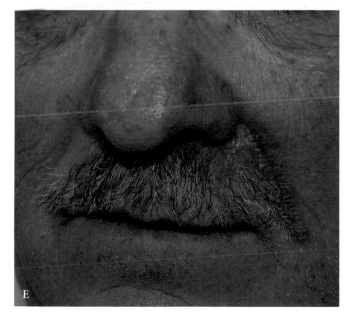

Figure 11.6 Rotation Flap.

A. Defect on the upper cutaneous lip bordering the melolabial fold. **B.** The flap incision is made along the melolabial fold in an arc shape and the dog-ear removed inferiorly in the radial relaxed skin tension line. **C.** The flap is draped into place pivoting around the oral commissure. **D.** Immediate post-op. **E.** Two weeks post-op. Note the symmetry in the position of the oral commissures.

(Continued on next page.)

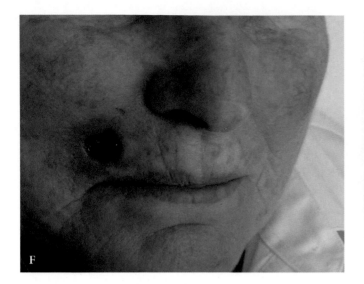

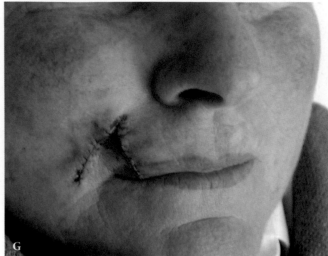

Figure 11.6 Rotation Flap *(continued).*

F. Defect that is more lateral and inferior. **G.** Incision made along the melolabial fold and dog-ear removed inferiorly along the RSTL extending through the vermilion border. **H.** Three years post-op. The placement of the incisions in naturally occurring creases and RSTL minimizes the visibility of the scar.

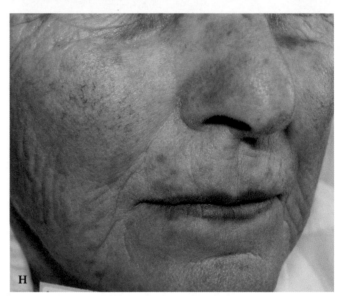

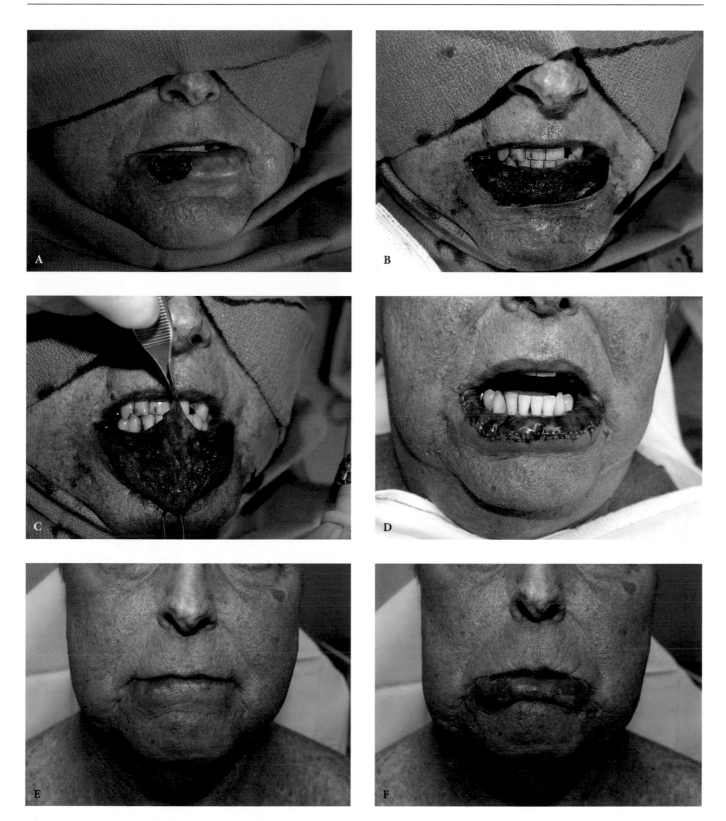

Figure 11.7 Mucosal Advancement Flap – Lower Lip.

A. Defect on the lower lip vermilion extending onto the skin. Mucosal advancement flaps are useful in replacing the entire vermilion lip when the orbicularis muscle is intact. **B.** Remainder of the vermilion is excised and the skin portion of the defect is tapered to blend bilaterally. **C.** The mucosa is undermined at the level of the minor salivary glands to the gingival sulcus. **D.** Immediate post-op. **E, F.** Five weeks post-op. Note that the lip is fully functional.

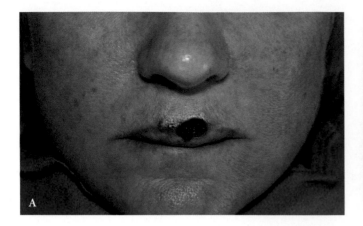

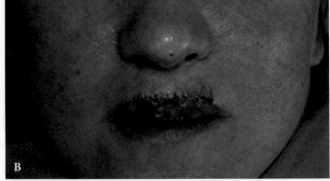

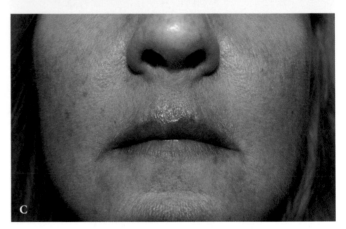

Figure 11.8 Mucosal Advancement Flap – Upper Lip.

A. Defect on the upper lip cupid's bow region involving both vermilion and skin. Reconstruction of the central upper lip must preserve the philtrum and cupid's bow. **B.** Immediate post-op. The mucosa is advanced and reapproximated with the skin along the vermilion border. **C.** Three months post-op. Note the preservation of the vermilion border and cupid's bow.

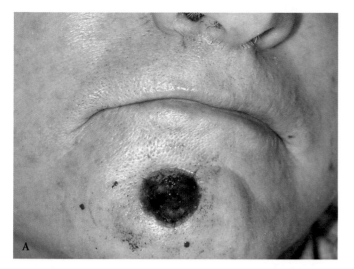

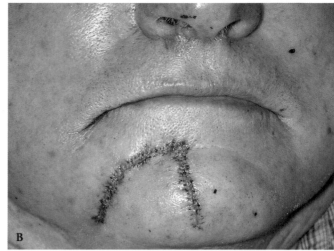

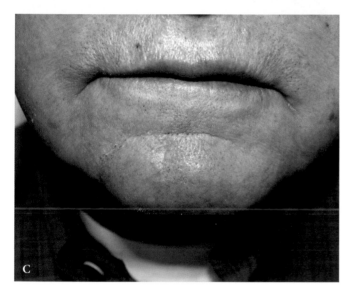

Figure 11.9 Rotation Flap.

A. Defect on the chin bordering the mental crease. Incisions on the chin should either be in the mental crease or vertically oriented. **B.** The flap incision is made along the mental crease arc. **C.** Two years post-op.

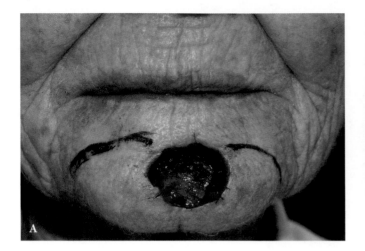

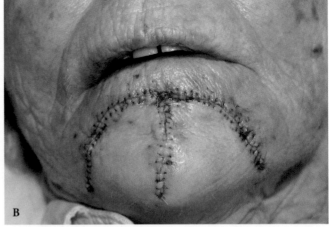

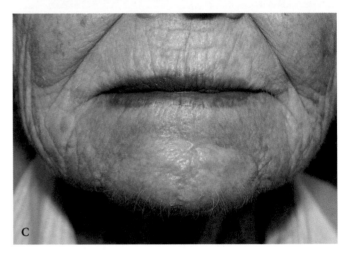

Figure 11.10 Bilateral Rotation Flap.

A. Defect on the central chin bordering the mental crease. **B.** Immediate post-op. Given the size, a bilateral rotation flap is needed with incisions along the mental crease arc. **C.** Two months post-op.

Index

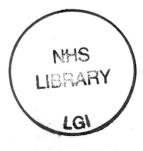